The Little
Psychotherapy Book

The Little Psychotherapy Book

Object Relations in Practice

ALLAN G. FRANKLAND, MD
Clinical Instructor, Department of Psychiatry
University of British Columbia
Staff Psychiatrist, Psychiatry Outpatient Department
Vancouver General Hospital
Vancouver, British Columbia, Canada

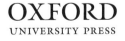

OXFORD

UNIVERSITY PRESS

2010

OXFORD
UNIVERSITY PRESS

Oxford University Press, Inc., publishes works that further
Oxford University's objective of excellence
in research, scholarship, and education.

Oxford   New York

Auckland   Cape Town   Dar es Salaam   Hong Kong   Karachi
Kuala Lumpur   Madrid   Melbourne   Mexico City   Nairobi
New Delhi   Shanghai   Taipei   Toronto

With offices in

Argentina   Austria   Brazil   Chile   Czech Republic   France   Greece
Guatemala   Hungary   Italy   Japan   Poland   Portugal   Singapore
South Korea   Switzerland   Thailand   Turkey   Ukraine   Vietnam

Published by Oxford University Press, Inc.
198 Madison Avenue, New York, New York 10016

www.oup.com

Oxford is a registered trademark of Oxford University Press

Library of Congress Cataloging-in-Publication Data
Frankland, Allan G.
The little psychotherapy book: object relations in practice / by Allan G. Frankland.
p. ; cm.
Includes bibliographical references and index.
ISBN 978-0-19-539081-0
1. Object relations (Psychoanalysis)   2. Psychodynamic psychotherapy.   I. Title.
[DNLM: 1. Object Attachment.   2. Professional—Patient
Relations.   3. Psychotherapy—methods. WM 460.5.O2 F831L 2010]
RC489.O25F73 2010
616.89′14—dc22
2009028234

Printed in the United States of America
on acid-free paper

To my daughter,
Lia Frankland

Acknowledgments

I would like to offer a few words of thanks to the people without whom this book would not have been possible. First, thank you to my friend and mentor, Dr. James Hillen, who spent countless hours explaining the mysteries of psychotherapy to me. Much of what I know about psychotherapy he taught me. I remember those Friday afternoons fondly! I would also like to thank Dr. Brian MacDonald and Dr. Leslie Flynn, each of whom played an important role in my development as a psychiatrist and therapist. I would also like to extend a hearty thanks to all of the residents and other colleagues who provided me with feedback about this book. Lastly, I would like to thank my wife (and best proofreader), Dr. Fia Voutsilakos.

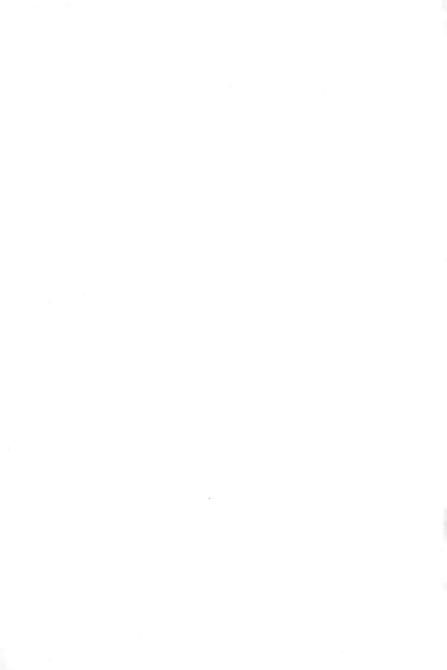

Contents

Contents

Contents

The Little
Psychotherapy Book

Introduction

The decision to write this book stemmed from my observation that many of the students I have worked with have expressed a desire to learn the basic nuts and bolts of how to perform psychodynamic psychotherapy from an object relations perspective. My aim is to provide clear and practical guidance to beginning therapists. I hope that this book will also be useful to more experienced therapists from other orientations who are seeking to develop an understanding of the day-to-day, practical application of object relations. I am hoping to answer the question: So how do you actually do it? Object relations therapy is complex, as are relationships in general. It is especially unfortunate that much of the literature about object relations is fraught with complicated terminology and concepts. Different terms often seem to have different meanings depending on the context and author. This makes learning object relations (especially from a book) particularly challenging.

My approach in writing this basic guide was to try to write a book that in retrospect would have been most useful to me during my training. I asked myself the following questions: What do I wish I had understood better when I was first starting out? What would be the simplest way to explain and illustrate the most important concepts and skills? How much information would be optimal for the beginning psychodynamic therapist? The result is a book that I hope:

- Promotes understanding while keeping complicated theory and terminology to a minimum
- Provides useful examples of the most common clinical situations
- Is concise—focusing specifically on the most important and practical material

There is a wise saying in the martial arts tradition: The best way to teach someone nothing is to teach him everything. I believe this to be true, particularly when trying to help someone develop a challenging new skill. Thus, this text is not intended to be an in-depth discussion of object relations history, theory, or terminology. Rather, I am hopeful that it will provide a starting point, a straightforward and practical how-to manual for interested students of psychodynamic psychotherapy—a group to which I also proudly belong. This text is intended to complement your training in psychotherapy. It would be a mistake to think that this (or any other book for that matter) could replace psychotherapy supervision and other forms of instruction. Also, at the end of the book is a glossary of key terms (that are in boldface throughout the text), as well as a list of titles I would recommend for further reading.

In many of the chapters I have included sample dialogues between Susan, a fictitious patient, and her therapist. For the sake of simplicity, I will use the female pronoun when discussing Susan's case, and whenever referring to patients.[1] The sample dialogues are intended to illustrate a particular concept or topic. They may give you an idea about how one might handle a particular situation, but they are not intended to be dogmatic. Clearly, there are many ways to approach almost any given issue.[2] In addition, there are numerous stylistic and contextual elements involved in the practice of psychotherapy. Indeed, a therapist always has a broad array of options available. This is one of the important themes to keep in mind as you go through this text. Ideally, I hope that reading through my suggestions will incite you to think about the issues that commonly arise in therapy and consider various ways of addressing these issues.

---

[1] You will notice that I use the term patient rather than today's more politically correct term client. I do this partly because it is the term I became accustomed to during my medical training, and partly because I believe it reflects my duty and responsibility to those in my care.

[2] This text is intended to provide an introduction to psychodynamic psychotherapy from a predominantly object relations perspective. However, I have also endeavored to incorporate useful concepts, principles, and tactics from other theoretical frameworks, ideally illustrating a balanced, integrated approach to psychodynamic psychotherapy.

CHAPTER ONE

So What Is Object Relations Anyway?

So what is **object relations**? **Object relations** is one of the four main theoretical models of **psychodynamic psychotherapy**. The other three are **self psychology**, **ego psychology**, and **attachment theory**. The term **object relations** itself can initially seem somewhat confusing. The relations part is easy enough to understand: it has to do with the patient's relationships—with herself and with others. But what is meant by the term **object**? And why is it called *object* instead of just *human* relations? The term **object** was coined by Sigmund Freud in 1905. The term is used to convey the fact that sometimes people do not perceive others as they really are, but rather as they imagine them to be. It is as if they are having a relationship with a two-dimensional fantasy object/person in their minds, rather than with a multidimensional real person. A real person has a mixture of both desirable and less desirable qualities. A fantasy **object** may be inaccurately viewed as "all good" or "all bad." It can even flip-flop rapidly between the two, depending on the circumstances. This fantasy **object** may be viewed as capable of fulfilling all of the patient's wants and needs (which can be thought of as seductive to the patient), while simultaneously appearing to withhold this goodness from the patient (which can be seen as rejecting). Thus, the **object** (often called the *bad* **object**) can be viewed as both seductive and rejecting, often at the same time. Each person's particular **object** fantasy prototypes are influenced by the tapestry of emotionally intense "good" and "bad" experiences that occur very early in life, even within the first year (Kernberg, 1992).

The following scenario involving initial romantic attraction offers a useful example of an **object** fantasy at work. A man at a social gathering sees an attractive woman from across a crowded room. He observes her appearance and body language from afar and develops an immediate impression of her. He sees her as a larger-than-life goddess-like figure who could unlock a life of everlasting happiness and/or unlimited sexual gratification for him. Our hero has thus imbued her with tremendous power and life-changing qualities. These qualities are clearly fantastical. *We* know that this woman likely has a mixture of desirable and less desirable personal qualities, just like anyone else. But to our hero, she is a magical being. It is understandable then, that when he walks over to introduce himself, he feels anxious, trips and falls in front of her, embarrassed. She giggles at his misfortune. He is mortified and escapes as quickly as possible, feeling hurt and rejected. This example illustrates the inaccuracy of the **object** in our hero's mind, as well as both the seductive and rejecting qualities with which he has imbued the woman. His anxiety grew out of an inaccurate perception of her. Inaccurate perceptions can unconsciously color verbal and nonverbal communication, influencing the course of specific interactions or even entire relationships. As time goes on, the partner's true qualities may reveal themselves, and the inaccuracy of the fantasy may become evident. It is thus perhaps not surprising that someone might be romantically involved, possibly for many years, before one day making the realization: "I don't think that I ever really knew Katie at all. It's as if I've been living with a stranger for the past 6 years." Therapy can help patients to see themselves and others more realistically. This can free our patients to have relationships with others as they really are, rather than as they imagine them to be.

How do these problems develop in the first place? Otto Kernberg, one of the modern pioneers of **object relations** theory, has postulated that children develop patterns in their views of themselves and others in response to affectively intense early experiences, typically involving the primary caregiver (Kernberg, 1992). These intense experiences may involve feelings of love or hate in response to satiation or deprivation of the child's needs by the caregiver. These intense early experiences are believed to influence the child's developing relationship templates through a type of emotional/experiential imprinting (Kernberg, 1984). It is believed that these extreme, affectively laden "all-good" or "all-bad" experiences can become overrepresented in the child's developing conceptualization of self and others. They reflect extreme and unusual situations, rather than day-to-day uneventful life. When the associated extreme, polarized views of self and others are carried forward into future relationships, distorted perceptions can result. The person can thereby develop a tendency to view herself and/or others as all good or all bad and experience the corresponding affects (intense love or hate) that were connected to the formative early experiences.

Advances in technology and research methodology have led to a growing body of neuroscientific and other evidence that is gradually confirming long-held psychodynamic theories and assumptions. Studies have demonstrated that early child–caregiver interactions have a significant impact on the developing brain (Chugani et al., 2001; Graham et al., 1999; Schore, 2001) and neurohormonal physiology (Ahnert et al., 2004; Anisman et al., 1998; Blunt Bugental et al., 2003; Hertsgaard et al., 1995; Gunnar et al., 1989; Ladd et al., 1996). These early interactions have known psychopathological correlates later in life (Beatson and Taryan, 2003; Graham et al., 1999; Raine et al., 2003; Sanchez et al., 2001). Early child–caregiver experiences combine with the child's various inherited dimensions of temperament to shape personality (Cloninger et al., 1993). Advances in the conceptualization of memory systems (Squire, 1987; Westen, 1999; Westen and Gabbard, 2002a, 2002b) have delineated unconscious forms of memory and memory retrieval that are involved in patterns of social relatedness, unconscious use of **defense mechanisms**,[1] and unconscious associations between present and past experiences (Gabbard, 2004, pp. 8–12). Psychotherapy has been shown to have an impact on the function (Etkin et al., 2005; Jung-Beeman et al., 2004), neurochemistry (Viinamaki et al., 1998), and neural networking (Gabbard and Westen, 2003) of the brain. It has also long been known that psychodynamic therapy improves quality of life (Piper et al., 1990; Shefler et al., 1995; Siegal et al., 1977; Sloane et al., 1975). However, this new wave of research is demonstrating

---

[1] **Defense mechanism**: a typically unconscious mental process that protects the individual from anxiety-provoking, unacceptable, or otherwise distressing psychic experiences. Please see the glossary for definitions of common **defense mechanisms**.

(e.g., via functional imaging) that psychotherapy also has a measurable and observable neurophysiological impact. With studies such as these, long-standing psychodynamic notions regarding the etiological mechanisms and treatment of psychopathology are gradually moving beyond theory, into the realm of empirical fact.

So how does therapy help address distorted perceptions of self and others, and the relationship difficulties that can ensue? This occurs by providing the patient with a new relationship experience that helps her to see herself and others more realistically, that is, as whole, multifaceted people, rather than simply as reflections of inaccurate internal fantasies. As **object relations** therapists, we use our experience of the therapeutic relationship in the here and now to guide and refine our understanding of the difficulties the patient has in relating to herself and others. Often, our emotional reactions provide us with some of the most important information about what is going on in the therapeutic relationship. As a result, this style of therapy can be emotionally charged for both patient and therapist. You may be wondering how the therapist decides what to say in all the different situations that can arise in therapy. The good news is that similar themes tend to arise repeatedly. I will discuss a number of recurring themes, as well as some suggestions to help you address them, in subsequent chapters. Once we understand what is going on between the patient and ourselves, we can then consider options for how to proceed. The most important thing to understand at this point, however, is that the therapeutic relationship itself is the template upon which change occurs in this style of therapy. In order to use that relationship to make helpful interventions, we must carefully observe our patients and ourselves. This requires thoughtful monitoring of one's emotional reaction to what is taking place.

CHAPTER TWO

The Big Picture

Having the big picture in mind is often very helpful when one is about to embark on a journey. Thus, I have included this section early in the text to give you an idea of what the "journey" of therapy may look like and of some possible areas of patient progress. We have already discussed a few of the issues that are commonly addressed in therapy. I do not think of therapy as a particularly linear process, with one stage necessarily preceding the next stage for completion. In my experience therapy tends to ebb and flow between various stages and issues. The dictum "a few steps forward and one step back" seems to hold true quite often. Nonetheless, the general areas of progress mentioned earlier have in my experience been remarkably similar for many of the patients I have worked with. This has led to my belief that people and their relationship difficulties tend to be more similar than different. I find this reassuring, as it suggests that it is possible to develop a solid foundation of understanding about human relationships in general. Once this foundation has been built, it becomes much easier to recognize and adapt to patients' individual differences.

So what are the possible areas of progress that patients can expect from long-term (i.e., over 24 sessions) **psychodynamic psychotherapy**? Below is a list of a number of potential benefits:

- Improving the quality of one's relationships
- Developing a defined and stable sense of self/identity
- Developing the capacity to observe one's thoughts, feelings, and behavior
- Developing one's ability to accurately conceptualize the emotional experience of others
- Developing awareness of one's internal psychological conflicts and how these intrapsychic conflicts can stir up anxiety and other distressing emotions
- Developing an awareness of one's **defense mechanisms**
- Developing healthier **defense mechanisms**
- Developing the ability to calm oneself down when distressed
- Developing a stable, balanced, and accurate mental image of others, even in their absence
- Developing the capacity to create and maintain appropriate relationship boundaries
- Shifting one's focus from negativity/self-criticism/frustration to focusing on positivity/self-acceptance/loving feelings
- Developing the capacity to accept and tolerate neediness in relationships, rather than attacking it or avoiding it
- Processing/grieving the damage that can result from negligent or abusive parenting

- Learning how to tolerate and manage imbalances (e.g., power imbalances) in relationships
- Processing and tolerating loss and relationship endings

Many of the benefits of psychotherapy occur through the experience of the unique qualities of the therapeutic relationship (Horvath and Symonds, 1991). Others may occur through specific and repeated therapeutic interventions. I would imagine that looking at this long list of areas of progress could seem a bit daunting. I would agree that there is a lot going on in therapy. Therefore, although it is important to be aware of the many dimensions along which change can occur, it is equally important to develop a core focus of treatment that is informed by your understanding of your particular patient (i.e., your formulation of the patient's core difficulty).[1] This brings us to one of the main features of **object relations** psychotherapy: its emphasis on understanding and addressing pathology within the patient's style of relating.

We must try to understand any repeated patterns of distortion in the patient's particular ways of viewing herself and others. These possibly inaccurate mental images of self and others are known as **self representations** and **object representations**, respectively. A thorough patient assessment can help one formulate an initial impression of any patterns with regard to these representations. Of course, one's understanding of such patterns is refined during

---

[1] In short-term treatments (i.e., fewer than 24 sessions) it is even more important to formulate and focus on a small number (perhaps one or two) of core treatment goals.

the course of therapy, largely through careful observation of what is taking place within the therapeutic relationship. This allows the therapist to observe and understand the problems as they arise in the moment, rather than rely solely on the patient's possibly distorted views and descriptions of problems in other relationships. Hence, **object relations** therapy tends to be very focused on the here and now of the therapeutic relationship.

A patient's tendency to see herself and others as either "all good" or "all bad" reflects significant distortions in her **self** and **object representations**. One of the particular strengths of **object relations** therapy lies in helping such patients develop a more balanced view of self and others that reflects the simultaneous existence of both good and bad qualities. This involves helping patients to see themselves and others as shades of gray, rather than just as black or white. Thus, one of the primary goals when treating patients with polarized, highly distorted **self** and **object representations** (a tendency known as **partial object relations**) should be to help them develop an integrated view of themselves and others (i.e., perceiving good and bad qualities as coexistent within the same individual). The capacity and tendency to adopt this type of integrated view is known as **whole object relations**. In order to accomplish this, the therapist must seek to identify and avoid engaging in pathological interaction styles, and respond in ways that promote awareness and integration of the polarized **self** and **object representations**. When these capacities have developed and are sustained over time, then the patient should be capable of experiencing healthier relationships that are based in reality, rather than fantasy.

CHAPTER THREE

Assessment and Formulation

How does one go about conducting an assessment that will help uncover the patient's relationship problems, determine suitability for psychotherapy, and guide psychotherapeutic treatment? I think the key is to perform an assessment interview that promotes a thorough understanding of your patient and her particular difficulties (i.e., your formulation). This understanding may be informed by an accurate DSM-IV-TR (American Psychiatric Association, 2000) diagnosis, but it should in fact be deeper and broader than that. Ideally, a psychodynamic therapist should seek to understand the potential biological, psychological, social, cultural, and spiritual factors that may contribute to the patient's problems. In addition, your assessment should identify whether the patient possesses some of the favorable characteristics believed to predict a good response to **psychodynamic psychotherapy**. Lastly, when specifically considering a course of **object relations** therapy, it is particularly important to try to uncover the patient's tendencies with regard to **self** and **object representations** and to determine whether the patient uses **partial** or **whole object relations** (as defined in the previous chapter).

How to go about doing all of this involves a sound approach to psychiatric interviewing. Psychiatric interviewing is a big topic, the details of which are beyond the scope of this book.[1] Therefore, I will assume that you are already familiar with the basic psychiatric interview and its various components. I would, however, like to suggest a mnemonic for a five-step approach to the assessment process that I believe will serve you well, both for interviewing and (with a couple of minor modifications) for conducting psychotherapy sessions.

In the first several minutes of the interview, it is typically prudent to listen to the patient's description of her concerns without prematurely attempting to focus the discussion (e.g., via early overuse of closed-ended questions). These first several minutes can be thought of as a scouting period, during which you are trying to get a sense of what the key issues are. When teaching interviewing skills, I will often suggest trying to accomplish "five things in the first five minutes." Figure 3.1 illustrates this approach.

Notice that the five key steps spell the acronym H.O.R.S.E. These five steps can provide guidance in interview situations and are also relevant to conducting psychotherapy (if you substitute the word

---

[1] I would refer you to Shawn Shea's book *Psychiatric Interviewing: The Art of Understanding* for a thorough review of this important aspect of clinical care.

THE H.O.R.S.E. INTERVIEWING APPROACH

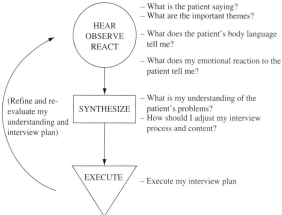

Figure 3.1 The H.O.R.S.E Interviewing Approach

"interview" in the graphic with "psychotherapy"). So remember, if you are struggling with a difficult interview or therapy session, you can depend on your trusty H.O.R.S.E. to carry you through it.

The first two parts of this approach ("hear" and "observe") may initially seem quite self-explanatory. However, as we will see in Chapter Eight (The Four Levels of Meaning), you can understand everything that the patient is communicating according to a number of different levels. Even deciphering what is being conveyed via body language is an art and a science in its own right.[2]

---

[2] I refer you to Barbara and Allan Pease's book *The Definitive Book of Body Language* and Paul Ekman's book *Emotions Revealed* (which unpacks facial expressions specifically).

You may be surprised by just how much one can surmise about a patient and her problems through careful observation of body language. It can be particularly revealing to observe and consider the context in which expressions of body language (e.g., facial expressions, gestures, posture, leg, foot, and arm positioning) change during an interview.

The "react" part of the H.O.R.S.E. approach involves paying careful attention to your own emotional reaction to the patient's behavior, speech content and style, and overall demeanor. This reaction is known as **countertransference**,[3] and it can reveal a wealth of information about the patient and her relationships. It is imperative that you pay close attention to this, both during your assessments and throughout each psychotherapy session. Ask yourself: What am I feeling? Am I feeling sad? Anxious? Irritated? Confused? Amused? Or perhaps some combination of these? What does this tell me about the patient? With practice this will become second nature to you and you will become more proficient at applying the information you glean to both your interviews and your psychotherapy sessions. This should also help you understand and relate to your patients more quickly, and with greater depth.

You may have noticed that the "synthesize" step has two components to it: synthesizing your understanding of the patient's difficulties, and synthesizing a corresponding interview plan. Your interview plan can be divided into interview process and interview content. Within the process of the interview it is helpful

---

[3] **Countertransference**: the therapist's total emotional reaction to the patient.

to consider both relationship issues (e.g., development of thera-peutic alliance/collaborative rapport, expressions of empathy, reassurance, and instillment of hope), and interview technique issues (e.g., the mix of open versus closed-ended questions, inter-view organization/prioritization, use of summaries, and transi-tions between the various sections of the interview). Interview content, on the other hand, pertains to what you ask about in each of the sections of the interview. Ideally, the choices you make with regard to the application of these process and content issues will be guided and further refined by your developing under-standing of the patient as the interview progresses.

Synthesizing an understanding/formulation of your patient and her difficulties involves putting together all of the informa-tion communicated through what you have heard, what you have observed, and your emotional reaction to what has transpired so far. This is typically a simpler task when all three lines of evidence converge. For example: the patient is describing depressive symp-tomatology, she appears despondent, she is demonstrating neu-rophysiological signs of depression, and you feel sad as you listen to her talk and observe her demeanor. The situation is typically more complicated when the three lines of evidence are divergent. For example: the patient is describing anxiety symptoms, she appears calm and cheerful, and you are feeling confused and irritated in response to your interaction with her. I think it is clear that in the second example, one must consider and explore a broader range of diagnostic and formulation possibilities to explain the divergent lines of evidence.

In addition, it is important to synthesize an understanding of the patient's difficulties with regard to the potential biological, psychological, social, cultural, and spiritual factors involved.

Understanding these factors and how they relate to mental health difficulties is another very broad topic that I will not attempt to cover here.[4] Suffice it to say that these aspects of your formulation are important, not only with regard to selecting the appropriate treatment for your patient but also to avoid overlooking important aspects of the patient's situation that could potentially be a primary or contributing cause of her problems (e.g., a medical condition that could cause or aggravate anxiety). For this reason, a history and physical examination (usually performed by the patient's primary care physician) and any appropriate investigations are also integral to the assessment process.

As we are talking about an assessment with a view to proposing **psychodynamic psychotherapy** as a treatment, it is also important to explore whether your patient possesses some of the characteristics that are believed to be associated with a good treatment outcome. These include a capacity for self-reflection, a capacity for abstract thought, an interest in self-understanding/introspection, and some capacity for frustration tolerance (Gabbard, 2004, p. 32). Lastly, since we are talking about performing therapy from a predominantly **object relations** perspective, it is particularly important to ask about the patient's history of relationships. Are there patterns in the way the patient tends to begin or end relationships? Do the patient's adult relationships seem to re-create aspects of her relationships with early caregivers? Or does she seem to go out of her way to form relationships that are the complete opposite of her early

---

[4] For further reading about this, please see Nancy McWilliams' book *Psychoanalytic Case Formulation* and Glen Gabbard's book *Psychodynamic Psychiatry in Clinical Practice.*

experiences? Additionally, it is useful to inquire about how the patient views herself, how she sees others, and how she believes others tend to view her. These lines of inquiry can help clarify the patient's **self** and **object representations**, and they can reveal whether the patient uses predominantly **partial** or **whole object relations**.[5] This last issue is especially important when developing a treatment plan for a course of **object relations** psychotherapy.

As was mentioned in the last chapter, individuals with **partial object relations** tend to see themselves and others as alternating between "all good" and "all bad" extremes. Thus, the primary treatment goal for individuals with **partial object relations** typically involves helping them to develop the capacity for a more balanced, integrated view of self and others. Secondary treatment goals might include developing the capacity for self-reflection, decreasing impulsivity, improving judgment, improving reality testing (Gabbard, 2004), and improving the patient's capacity to maintain a stable, balanced, and accurate mental representation of others (including the therapist) in their absence (known as **object constancy**—a term coined by Heinz Hartmann in 1952).

By contrast, individuals with **whole object relations** already tend to see themselves and others in a balanced and integrated way. Despite this, such individuals may still experience internal conflicts that can cause them distress and relationship difficulties. These intrapsychic conflicts often result in anxiety that can

---

[5] **Partial** versus **whole object relations** are concepts that are also relevant to distinguishing between **borderline** and **neurotic personality organization**. For more about these constructs, please see Glen Gabbard's book *Long-Term Psychodynamic Psychotherapy: A Basic Text*, p. 31.

manifest in various ways. These manifestations of anxiety are colored by the individual's use of **defense mechanisms**, which may be conscious, unconscious, useful and healthy (often classified as "mature"), or unhealthy and problematic (often classified as "immature").[6] In patients who use **whole object relations**, the primary goal of therapy would typically involve helping the patient to explore and consciously understand her intrapsychic conflicts as they are enacted within the therapeutic relationship. As this process of exploration is repeated over time, these conflicts typically become less anxiety provoking and problematic to the patient. Additional goals might include improving anxiety management and helping the patient shift toward use of predominantly healthy **defense mechanisms**.

---

[6] A third grouping of **defense mechanisms** (known as "neurotic" **defense mechanisms**) forms a "middle zone of maturity" between the immature and mature defenses. These defenses are commonly employed by individuals with **neurotic personality organization**.

CHAPTER FOUR

Patient Selection: Susan's Case

In this chapter, I will describe the assessment of a fictitious patient named Susan, to whom I will refer frequently throughout the rest of the text. I will then review the formulation of her case and the corresponding treatment plan with respect to psychotherapy. In addition, I will be discussing some additional suggestions for selecting appropriate patients when seeking to develop some initial experience with **object relations** therapy. The following is a description of Susan's assessment.

On the day of her assessment interview, Susan presents approximately 10 minutes early for her appointment. She has been referred by her family doctor for diagnostic clarification and for assessment regarding her request for psychotherapy. After the initial introductions, the interviewer asks Susan about her understanding of the reason for referral and subsequently about what she herself is hoping to address (as these often differ). The interviewer then allows Susan to describe her concerns freely for several minutes. The interviewer listens carefully, observes her facial expressions, body language, and demeanor, and monitors for any particular emotional reactions to her. During these first several minutes, the interviewer asks few questions and instead prompts Susan to continue talking about her primary concerns. This is accomplished using phrases such as: "Please go on," "What happened next?" and "Can you tell me more?"

Susan explains that she is a 25-year-old single woman who lives alone in an apartment. She has been working as a clerical office assistant at a law firm for the past 6 months. The main themes of her presenting concerns are as follows: Susan states that she has been chronically unhappy and dissatisfied with her life. She describes longstanding difficulties with self-esteem, self-criticism, and a tendency toward pessimism. She has always been easily moved to irritation or anxiety in response to day-to-day situational stress in her workplace interactions, friendships, and romantic relationships. Currently, she is frustrated with her employer, whom she describes as "nothing but a slave-driver." She also notes dissatisfaction with her new romantic relationship, describing her new boyfriend Jeff as "distant." With regard to previous boyfriends, she states that they have either been annoyingly distant or overly controlling. She also wonders whether she might have a tendency to "sabotage relationships somehow," perhaps leading others to mistreat her. Susan indicates that she tends to be quite sensitive to others' comments about her. She has noticed only slightly decreased anxiety over the past 2 years, since agreeing to her family physician's suggestion that she try an antidepressant. She describes a keen interest in individual therapy to cope better with stress, understand herself better, and sort out her relationship difficulties.

Although these are the key points that Susan discusses in the first several minutes of free speech, she presents the issues in a disjointed and convoluted manner. She often jumps from topic to topic and provides few contextual details. She appears to be growing unsettled and somewhat irritated by the lack of guidance from the interviewer.

Susan is well dressed and groomed. The interviewer notes no overt manifestations of neurophysiological symptoms of depression (such as psychomotor slowing/lethargy, quiet or slowed speech, slumped posture, downcast gaze, or concentration difficulties). Susan appears comfortable as she sits with her legs crossed, gesticulating frequently with her hands (typically with palms facing upward toward the ceiling—which the interviewer notes as an indication that she is trying to be open and honest). Her affect appears to fluctuate from calm and euthymic to transiently dysphoric and irritated, depending on what she is talking about. She appears neither pervasively sad nor anxious.

On a couple of occasions the interviewer notes feeling somewhat irritated, perhaps in reaction to Susan's tendency to provide a convoluted, disorganized description of her difficulties. After about 5 minutes, the interviewer summarizes the key themes that Susan has described. Susan folds her arms in front of her before listening to this brief summary. The interviewer mentally notes Susan's shift to a closed posture. The interviewer then asks whether Susan has been feeling frustrated about the various difficulties she has described. Susan agrees, uncrosses her arms, and leans forward ever so slightly in her seat. The interviewer remarks, "Susan at this point I'd like to ask you some specific questions about the difficulties you've described." The interviewer hopes and expects that a shift to a more directive interviewing approach involving more specific questions will help ease Susan's irritation and promote clearer responses.

The interviewer asks some questions to clarify Susan's mood and anxiety symptoms. This leads to a feeling of confusion (adding to the interviewer's previously noted irritation) as Susan continues to answer these more focused questions in a rather vague and convoluted way. However, there is no evidence of formal thought disorder that might be suggestive of a psychotic process. She endorses some of the symptoms of depression, as well as some symptoms of anxiety. These symptoms do not clearly meet the threshold for a diagnosis of a specific anxiety or depressive disorder, however. Her anxiety and depressive symptoms are reportedly transient and tend to occur primarily in the context of interpersonal tension. The interviewer wonders how to piece together the available information into a cohesive initial understanding of Susan and her difficulties.

Susan's presentation is neither predominately sad nor predominately anxious. The emotional reactions that she is engendering seem to be confusion and irritability as opposed to sadness or anxiety. The interviewer wonders whether the diverging lines of evidence in Susan's endorsed symptoms, demeanor, as well as the emotional responses she seems to be triggering, may in fact be suggestive of interpersonal difficulties that may be unrelated (or perhaps only peripherally related) to any specific mood or anxiety disorder.

The interviewer attempts to politely refocus Susan's circumstantial responses several times. On these occasions Susan tends to cross her arms in front of her and lean back in her seat. On one of these instances, the interviewer mentions: "I realize that I've been asking you a lot of difficult questions today, Susan. I wonder how you're doing at this point?" Susan responds by saying: "I'm a little irritated that you keep interrupting me . . . but I guess you're just doing your job." The interviewer wonders whether this may represent evidence of a capacity for **mentalization**. In other words, Susan may have some ability to reflect on her own mental/emotional state and simultaneously put herself "in someone else's shoes."

The interviewer screens for current and past safety issues. Susan states that she has experienced vague suicidal ideation that "life isn't worth it" on rare occasions when very distressed (e.g., in response to tension with her employer or in the context of romantic difficulties) in the past, but she states that this has never progressed to suicidal intent or planning. She reports no current or recent difficulties with suicidal ideation or self-harm behavior. She mentions that she had cut her arm superficially on impulse once during her late teens, after a relationship breakup. The interviewer also performs screens for alcohol and recreational drug overuse, eating disorder symptoms, and psychotic symptoms, all of which are negative. The interviewer then summarizes some of the key findings of the history of presenting illness before transitioning to past history. Susan reveals that she has had no prior history of mental health contacts or treatments. She is physically healthy and takes only the antidepressant prescribed by her family physician. There is no family history of diagnosed mental illness or of attempted or completed suicide. The interviewer then reviews Susan's personal and developmental history, including Susan's recollection of her childhood, developmental milestones, her relationship with each of her parents, her experience of school, her work history, and her history of friendships and romantic relationships.

Susan describes a lifelong intact yet tense relationship with her mother. She remarks that her mother "has always been critical and controlling" and adds that she would often "fly off the handle," yelling at Susan or her father. When asked, Susan is unable to identify or describe any of her mother's positive qualities. Susan goes on to state that she wonders whether her relationship with her mother may have been emotionally abusive. The interviewer then asks Susan about her relationship with her father, whom she states "wasn't really there" for her during her childhood and teenage years. The interviewer reflects that it must have been challenging for Susan to grow up in her household, given the difficult relationships she has described. The interviewer decides to see how Susan will respond to an **interpretation** identifying a parallel between her experience of the interviewer in the here and now and her relationship with her mother: "You mentioned earlier feeling irritated by some of my interruptions. I wonder if to some extent you've experienced me today as trying to control you, perhaps like you said your mother did growing up?" Susan thinks about this for a moment before answering that she has always been sensitive to people trying to control her, particularly in the workplace and within romantic relationships.

Susan indicates that she moved out of the family home at the age of 19 to escape tension in the household. She denies any history of physical or sexual abuse. She states that she did well academically and enjoyed school as an escape from her rather tense home life. After graduating high school she began clerical office work. She indicates that she has kept most of her jobs for between 6 and 12 months before frustrations involving either co-workers or employers have led her to give notice and find work elsewhere. She has never walked off the job or quit impulsively. She has never been fired. She left her last job due to feeling disliked and criticized by her employer.

4. Patient Selection: Susan's Case

Susan describes a history of difficulties maintaining friendships and romantic relationships, adding that she will sometimes "cut people out" of her life if they disappoint or betray her. When asked about which personal qualities she likes about herself, she states that she will "go all out" to help a friend in need. She adds that she feels disappointed when her friends do not reciprocate to the same degree when she is in need of assistance. When asked which of her personal qualities she finds less appealing, she describes being "too sensitive." Regarding how she views others, Susan indicates that she finds it "hard to really trust people." In terms of how she believes others view her, Susan states that she is unsure but thinks others probably see her as "really caring but maybe too sensitive."

As the interview draws to a close, the interviewer briefly summarizes some of the key issues that Susan has described and thanks her for her candor. The interviewer then ends on a hopeful note by commenting on Susan's resiliency despite difficulties in her early home life, as well as challenges within her personal and work relationships. The two then discuss a mutually agreeable time to meet again to discuss some issues related to treatment, including the possibility of individual psychotherapy.

Susan's history and presentation are most consistent with a DSM-IV-TR (American Psychiatric Association, 2000) diagnosis of depressive disorder not otherwise specified, possibly recurrent brief depressive disorder or dysthymic disorder. It is also possible that her depressive symptomatology may in fact be reflective of the impact of characterological difficulties on her mood. Susan's history and presentation do not appear suggestive of a personality disorder per se. She describes difficulties with emotion dysregulation, anger dyscontrol, and interpersonally based anxiety that appear episodic, rather than pervasive. Susan appears to function

29

quite well until faced with challenging interpersonal issues, which lead her to experience irritation, distress, and anxiety. These difficulties seem to reflect a transient, stress-related regression to a more primitive interaction style. At these times Susan seems to experience a pattern of **self** and **object representations** in which she views herself much like a resentful, victimized child, and others (often attachment or authority figures) as vindictive and controlling (much like her description of her mother). At other times she seems to view herself as a yearning and resentful child, while viewing attachment figures as passive and distant (much like her view of her father). Susan's **self** and **object representations** in both instances appear to be connected to each other by the affect of anger.[1] Her problematic relationship patterns appear to have their beginnings in her early caregiver relationships. Aspects of these early relationships seem to re-create themselves in her romantic and work relationships.

Susan seems to have some capacity for self-reflection/**mentalization**. She also describes a keen interest in self-understanding, and she has remained active in the workforce despite her difficulties. She does not endorse complicating comorbidities, such as recreational drug use or significant medical problems that could preclude regular attendance at psychotherapy sessions. As Susan has a tendency toward **partial object relations** (particularly when distressed in the context of attachment relationships), one of the primary treatment goals would be to help Susan develop more

---

[1] The **self representation**, the **object representation**, and the affect experienced regarding these representations together comprise an **object relations unit** (Kernberg, 1976, 1984).

accurate and integrated **self** and **object representations**. Secondary treatment goals might include further development of her capacity for self-reflection/**mentalization** and improvement in her management of intense emotions, particularly in the context of attachment relationships.

Selecting appropriate patients to engage in any type of therapy is clearly a very important initial step. This is particularly the case when selecting appropriate patients for a budding therapist who is trying to develop proficiency at **psychodynamic psychotherapy**. When first starting out, I would suggest beginning with a patient who experiences mild interpersonal pathology. There is enough to learn without having to manage more complicated and distressing issues such as serious self-harm or suicide attempts. An appropriate first patient might be someone in her[2] middle or late twenties (when characterological traits could still be expected to be quite fluid) who has maintained a few fairly stable relationships. She may have engaged in mild self-harm (e.g., superficial cutting) once or twice in the distant past but has never required hospitalization. She has never made a serious attempt to end her life and does not describe ongoing suicidal ideation. Thus, she is generally "safe and contained" prior to beginning therapy. Perhaps she has been working at the same job for many years. This may be somebody with some awareness that she tends to "create problems in relationships somehow" (an indicator of psychological mindedness), or that she tends to pick unsuitable romantic partners—perhaps partners who turn out to be emotionally distant, rather

---

[2] Reminder: I am still using the female pronoun solely for writing simplicity.

than physically abusive. Ideally, the patient would be capable of abstract thought and would already have demonstrated the capacity to tolerate some anxiety and frustration in her life without significant decompensation. Perhaps the patient has a DSM-IV-TR (American Psychiatric Association, 2000) diagnosis of dysthymic disorder, depressive disorder not otherwise specified, or anxiety disorder not otherwise specified. Ideally, this would be someone who describes a keen interest in understanding herself better through individual therapy and whose work schedule could accommodate regular weekly or twice weekly appointments. Get the idea? I am talking about somebody who is generally functioning quite well and already has some meaningful relationships. I am not talking about a person with a severe or even moderately severe personality disorder. I am certainly not talking about somebody who has had several admissions to hospital with multiple recent overdoses, or someone who has been on disability for several years. These more complicated patients would benefit from follow-up with somebody who already has a solid understanding of **object relations** principles and can use this understanding to adapt to the complexities involved in treating particularly challenging and potentially unstable patients. In addition, patients with significant comorbid substance use problems, acute mania, acute psychosis, or significant antisocial personality traits would likely not be appropriate candidates for this type of therapy.[3]

---

[3] While patients with such difficulties may not be suitable therapy candidates for the beginning **object relations** therapist, familiarity with **object relations** concepts and techniques could certainly inform and likely benefit their general treatment.

4. Patient Selection: Susan's Case

Okay, so let's say you have found somebody similar to the description above—ideally someone who experiences difficulties rooted in the interpersonal realm, is "safe and contained," has some capacity for self-reflection, is interested in pursuing therapy with you, is generally functioning quite well, and is in a life situation conducive to committing to regular weekly sessions. What next?

CHAPTER FIVE

The Treatment Contract

Once you have performed the initial assessment, determined that the patient is suitable for individual therapy, and formulated a treatment plan, the next steps will involve obtaining informed consent and establishing a (usually verbal) treatment contract. I would suggest at least one separate appointment to address these issues. During this appointment, I will usually describe "what therapy looks like." For example, I will explain: "We would be meeting once per week for 50 minutes. During that time we can talk about whatever you like, or, if you don't feel like talking, that's okay too." This statement may create some anxiety in the patient who may now be imagining sitting across from me in awkward silence for 50 minutes. If the person seems to be getting anxious about this, I will often make a reassuring statement. For example, I might say: "That may sound kind of stressful, but I suspect you will settle into it just fine. And I'll be here to help you along if need be." The topic of the anxiety and stress of therapy leads into a discussion of potential risks. I may say: "Therapy *is* a new kind of relationship and any change can be a little stressful. Because of that, once in a while people can initially feel like therapy is making them feel more upset or distressed. That's a risk that's important to understand. We can both watch out for that, and we can certainly work through it together if that happens, but I am expecting that you will adjust to therapy just fine. I wouldn't be suggesting it for you otherwise." I think it is important to explain the risk of deterioration honestly and clearly. I also think it is appropriate to give reassurance at this point to a patient whom you have already determined to be a good therapy candidate, and who is likely to derive significant benefit.

Notice that I said that the appointment would be "50 minutes." I did not say "around 50 minutes" or "just under an hour." I gave an exact duration. This is not a coincidence. This conveys a few different messages to the patient. The statement emphasizes that therapy will be structured and organized by the therapist. The power differential between therapist and patient is implicit in the statement, and many patients will notice or even react to this. The other message in the statement is: "I, the therapist, am in control." This metacommunication may sound somewhat authoritarian. However, it can be a reassuring message for patients who may spend much of the time feeling "out of control." It is also very clear that your time with the patient will be limited. Perhaps you are beginning to see the layers of complexity and meaning involved, even in one's choice of words. Please do not be intimidated by this. There is not an absolute "right" or "wrong" way of doing or saying things in therapy. Even if you later decide that another approach would have been preferable in a given situation, there are few things that you could say that would be impossible to redress, for example, during a subsequent session.

Next, I will usually describe my expectations of the patient. I will often say something like: "This type of therapy doesn't involve any homework, but I do ask a few things of you. It is important that you come to every appointment, and that you are on time. If something urgent comes up and you are unable to attend, I would ask that you please call and speak with me directly with as much advance notice as possible." This would also be an appropriate time to discuss any billing issues or expectations, if this is relevant to your practice situation.

Perhaps my expectations sound somewhat demanding and rigid. I am indeed creating a high expectation for the patient to attend "every appointment" in a punctual manner. Some patients may be surprised by this as well. But what does this convey to the patient? It says: "Your attendance in therapy is important to me and therapy should take a high priority in your life." If this is not easy to see initially, consider what would be conveyed by a very different statement: "This type of therapy doesn't involve any homework, and I don't mind much if you miss appointments or if you're late." Can you see that this second statement gives the impression that you do not really care? The therapist's creation of expectations, boundaries, and rules serves many functions, not the least of which is conveying concern for the patient's therapeutic progress. Patients will react to this in varying ways, and this has to do in part with the patient's reaction to your expression of neediness ("I need you to be here every week"). Your clear statement of the "rules of therapy" also highlights the power imbalance in the therapeutic relationship. *You* are the one creating the rules, *not* the patient. The patient's feelings about the imbalance of power are connected to the issue of neediness just mentioned. These issues tend to come up frequently in therapy as well as in relationships in general. How these issues intersect and how to address them will be discussed further in an upcoming chapter about neediness.

The elements of the treatment contract discussed above should be adequate for the therapy candidates that I have suggested selecting early on. Patients with more complicated difficulties may require additional elements in the treatment contract. These elements may include an agreement between the therapist and patient regarding other issues that could potentially threaten the treatment. The following are a few examples of potential therapy-interfering issues: preoccupation with procuring support and advice regarding day-to-day issues and decisions (rather than seeking to better understand one's internal world), recurrent suicidal threats and self-harm behaviors, grossly disordered eating patterns, and problematic substance abuse. Although such issues do not preclude psychotherapy by an experienced practitioner, patients with issues such as these would likely not be the most suitable candidates for new therapists who are seeking to develop proficiency in **object relations**–based therapy.[1]

---

[1] I refer you to *A Primer of Transference-Focused Psychotherapy for the Borderline Patient* (by Frank Yeomans, John Clarkin, and Otto Kernberg) for further reading regarding a more involved treatment contract for potentially unstable patients with more severe pathology (pp. 71–103).

CHAPTER SIX

The Value of Rules and Boundaries

In the last chapter, we saw an example of how the therapist's creation of expectations, rules, and boundaries regarding therapy can convey that he or she cares about the patient and her therapeutic progress. Let's look at another example to help illustrate the value of rules and boundaries in therapy. Imagine that our fictitious patient Susan is just about to begin psychotherapy with you. You have just met with her to discuss the therapeutic contract and what therapy will involve. You are now in the midst of discussing a mutually agreeable time to meet.

Susan: "So when do we actually start?"

Therapist: "Well, we will need to find a regular day and time that works for both of us."

Susan: "What would be best for me is to meet on Friday evenings at about 7 p.m. Can you meet then?"

Therapist: "That actually wouldn't work for me since my last appointment of the day is at 5 p.m. How would Thursdays at 2 p.m. work for you?"

Susan: "No that's no good for me—it would really cut up my day. How about 6 p.m. on Thursday? I could come straight here after my photography class—that way it would be so much more convenient."

How would you deal with this situation? Situations like this are not uncommon. You have not even started your first "official" session with this patient, yet therapy has clearly already begun. Let's consider what would be conveyed to the patient if you do not maintain firm boundaries in this situation. I would argue that failing to do so could potentially sabotage therapy with this patient in at least two ways. First, by making an exception for this patient, perhaps in the name of being a "good, caring, and accommodating therapist," you would in fact be demonstrating an inability to maintain boundaries that you yourself had introduced, that is, not seeing patients after 5 p.m. What might this convey to a patient who has difficulties creating or maintaining boundaries? Well, if she cannot form boundaries for herself, and you have just demonstrated that you cannot maintain your boundaries in the therapeutic relationship, then who will? The answer could be *nobody*! What a terrifying notion for a patient about to embark on the journey of therapy with you. It is as though you have agreed to be the captain of the sailing trip and you have just informed the patient that the boat has no rudder and you have no idea how to navigate. The patient should rightfully expect to be adrift at sea with you! A therapist who does not maintain boundaries can be very unsettling for patients. The second issue to consider is the possible effect of changing your normal routine on your attitude toward this patient and her therapy. As an example, perhaps extending your day by 1 hour leads you to be caught in a lengthy (e.g., 2 hour) commute home, whereas leaving 1 hour earlier avoids this. It is quite plausible that you might develop resentment about this and that you might, perhaps unconsciously, act out this resentment during the course of your patient's therapy. This would be an example of **negative countertransference**.[1] Therapy can thus effectively be contaminated or poisoned by an initial lack of boundaries. Indeed, making the sometimes difficult decision to maintain firm boundaries in the therapeutic relationship protects therapy from problems like those described above.

---

[1] **Negative countertransference** is a therapy-contaminating emotional reaction (in the therapist) to the patient that occurs as a result of the therapist's personal issues or needs.

CHAPTER SEVEN

Beginning the First Session

I have typically met the patient a few times prior to the first actual therapy session. On the day of the first session, I usually greet the patient in the waiting room (I work in a hospital-based outpatient psychiatry department) and invite her to my office. My typical greeting is very simple, for example, "Hi Susan, please come in." Particularly during the early stages of therapy, many patients will try to engage in small talk during the short walk to my office. I am typically polite and pleasant in this situation, but I do not tend to engage in lengthy conversations. Probably the most common question people ask at this point is: "How are you doing today?" I will typically respond that I am doing well. I may thank her for asking. I will not, however, ask how the patient is doing at that point. Remember, we are walking to my office. The patient's current emotional state is an important part of the therapy session and is thus best addressed once we are inside my office. It can seem somewhat unnatural initially not to reciprocate with: "I'm fine thanks, how are you?" My decision to minimize friendly chitchat prior to beginning the session is a conscious and important one. One of the common (typically unconscious) reasons that patients will seek to engage in friendly chitchat at this point is to decrease anxiety. Chitchat serves to create the illusion of a friendly, casual conversation and relationship. This can decrease the patient's anxiety by creating the illusion of a more even balance of power in the relationship. However, the therapist–patient relationship is neither a friendship nor a casual relationship. Rather, it is a uniquely personal yet still professional relationship. There *is* an imbalance of power in this relationship. To collude with the patient in conducting or portraying the relationship otherwise (e.g., as a chat between friends) is inaccurate and therefore does not serve the patient. Doing so would overlook the significant power imbalance issues in the relationship and the effects of these on the patient. Comments that serve to level the playing field in therapy are common reactions to the patient's perception and recognition of the power imbalance. This is an important issue that must not be swept under the carpet, but instead should be explicitly addressed in therapy. Power imbalances exist in many relationships, and how the patient deals with these issues will affect her ability to create and maintain healthy relationships in general.

Once we are seated in my office, I will typically write the person's name, the date, and the time of the appointment at the top of my notepad, and wait silently and intently. This may seem quite unnatural and uncomfortable to you initially. Once again, this initial silence is a conscious and important choice. (With very impaired patients, I may choose not to begin with silence, in order to provide ample structure to ease anxiety.[1] However, this is quite a different patient population than the patients I have suggested selecting early on, while you are first learning **psychodynamic psychotherapy**.) Remember how I suggested describing therapy to the patient in Chapter Five? I stated that the patient could talk about whatever she wanted, and if she did not want to talk, that would be all right as well. This cannot occur if I initiate the appointment with a question, effectively imposing my agenda on the session. Your initial silence provides the patient with the freedom to talk about whatever is on her mind.

Starting the session with silence may lead to some anxiety early on. I would suggest to you that our patients must experience *some* anxiety, as this provides an impetus for therapeutic change to take place. Thus, it is important to avoid providing too much structure or guidance, as this may lower the patient's anxiety level below the threshold needed to incite change. On the other hand, it is equally important to provide *enough* structure, guidance, and reassurance during the session to prevent the patient from becoming overwhelmed with anxiety. If patients become too distressed, they may decompensate, regress, and/or drop out of therapy altogether. As an example, the following brief exchange could occur in the first few moments of Susan's first therapy session:

Susan: (Initially silent, appears somewhat anxious, looking around the room for several seconds before speaking.) "I'm not really sure what to talk about . . . " (Smiles faintly.)

---

[1] We will discuss this concept further in Chapter Fifteen: Structure and How to Use It Therapeutically.

Therapist: "We can talk about whatever you'd like. If you don't have anything in particular to say, that's okay too. This is your time."

The therapist could respond in many different ways depending on how anxious Susan seems. If Susan does not seem very anxious at all, the therapist may choose not to respond to her comment at all, and to simply remain silent and allow her to continue when she is ready. At the other end of the spectrum, if Susan appears *very* anxious, the therapist may decide to provide even more structure and guidance than in the example. For instance, the therapist could respond by suggesting a topic to discuss: "Maybe you can start by telling me about your week." In general, I would try to avoid providing this much guidance and structure if at all possible, for the reasons already described. Another way to ease anxiety would be to engage the patient in describing her affect state. The following dialogue demonstrates this important technique:

Therapist: "You seem a little anxious . . . tell me all about how you're feeling right now."
Susan: "Well, I feel anxious, like you said."
Therapist: "Maybe you can start by telling me where you feel the anxiety in your body?"
Susan: "I kind of feel butterflies in my stomach . . ."
Therapist: "I see. What else do you feel physically?"
Susan: "Well, my muscles seem kind of tense and my hands are clenched."
Therapist: (Noticing that Susan already seems calmer.) "You seem a little more relaxed now."
Susan: "Yeah, I guess I am."

In the above dialogue, the therapist is asking Susan to observe and describe her affect state. Many patients struggle with observing and describing affect states, particularly if they are new to psychotherapy. The development of these skills is an important part of the therapeutic process. I have found the following three-step approach to be helpful for patients who may be struggling with this. In the first step, I will ask the patient to describe how the emotion is affecting her *physically*. Most patients find this to be the easiest step in the process. If this does not effectively decrease the intensity of the patient's affect, I will then ask the patient to describe her *thoughts* about the feeling or the relevant situation. Many patients find the final step—describing the emotion in *abstract* terms (e.g., using metaphors or similes)—to be the most challenging part of the process. Thus, I will often leave this step for last, once the patient has already calmed herself down somewhat through the first two steps. At each step along the way, I encourage the patient to be as detailed as possible: "Try to paint a picture of it for me with your words, using as much detail as you can." Why do you think this technique is effective for helping patients to calm down and reduce the intensity of their emotions? Well, a big part of it has to do with engaging the aspect of one's mind that observes oneself (coined the **observing ego** by Sigmund Freud in 1933). Due to the limited capacity and selective nature of attention, it is very difficult for the human mind to focus on more than one task at a time (Abernethy, 1988; Guttentag, 1989). If we can help our patients to become immersed in observing and describing their affect states, it becomes more difficult for them to remain overwhelmed and carried away by the intensity of their emotions. Thus, the very act of observing oneself in detail helps calm people down and helps reduce the intensity of whatever emotion

45

they are experiencing. This technique is amazingly effective.[2] Once patients have practiced this enough with you, they can begin to observe their affect on their own in other situations as well. Often, the most difficult part can be helping particularly challenging or particularly distressed patients to actually engage in the process to begin with.

---

[2] In Chapter Eleven (Anxiety and the Paranoid-Schizoid Position) we will be reviewing a dialogue that illustrates this three-step technique in more detail.

CHAPTER EIGHT

The Four Levels of Meaning

Beginning therapists often wonder how to understand what is being communicated by the patient. The H.O.R.S.E. approach presented in Chapter Three (Assessment and Formulation) can be very useful in this regard. Figure 8.1 illustrates the H.O.R.S.E. approach adapted for psychotherapy.

Using this approach, I would consider the three lines of information (i.e., what I hear, what I observe, and my emotional reaction) about a situation in order to synthesize a provisional understanding of what is going on in the exchange. I would then use this understanding to help decide what to say next. This may sound like a complicated process to use, just to determine what to say. Indeed, this is a skill that develops with a lot of practice, supervision, and time spent considering what happened—usually in retrospect, after the session is over. As I had mentioned in an earlier chapter, however, the themes that arise in therapy are often surprisingly similar from person to person. Thus, one develops a

THE H.O.R.S.E. PSYCHOTHERAPY APPROACH

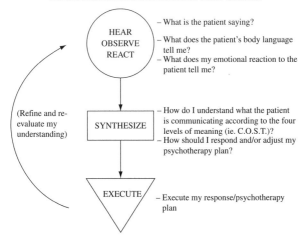

Figure 8.1 The H.O.R.S.E Psychotherapy Approach

familiarity with addressing the common themes and adapting one's responses to the particular patient and situation. This is a process of continual learning. It is one of the challenges that makes conducting therapy so stimulating and rewarding.

In this chapter, I would like to offer an easy-to-remember approach that can help you synthesize your understanding of inter-actions (i.e., the "S" part of H.O.R.S.E.) during your sessions, according to the four possible levels of meaning referred to in the H.O.R.S.E. graphic. So what are the four levels of meaning? To help illustrate the four levels, let's first consider another sample dialogue with Susan, our fictitious patient, who has recently started therapy and is describing her relationship with her new boyfriend.

(Therapist and patient both sit down to begin the therapy session. Therapist is silent.)

Susan: "So I've just started dating this guy named Jeff, and I'm not sure where it's going to go . . ."

Therapist: (Silent, listening.)

Susan: "I bet he's going to end up being cold and distant like most of my exes. That wouldn't surprise me. He already kind of seems that way."

Therapist: "It sounds as if you feel some uncertainty about this new relationship and where it might be going . . . tell me what that's like for you."

Susan: "Well, he's just kind of quiet and he really doesn't talk much. But I suppose I should be used to it by now. My boyfriends always turn out to be either cold and distant or totally intense and controlling. There doesn't seem to be anything I can do about it." (Spoken with an irritated tone.)

Therapist: "You seem irritated, even now as you talk about it. Tell me all about what you are feeling right now."

Susan: "Really? I wasn't really aware of feeling anything, but now that you mention it, maybe I am feeling kind of annoyed."

When synthesizing an understanding of this exchange, it can be helpful to think in terms of the four levels of meaning illustrated in Figure 8.2.[1]

---

[1] Please note: the "four levels of meaning" are not "official" **object relations** theory per se. Rather, this is a framework (adapted from teaching passed on to me by my psychotherapy supervisor) for a useful approach to decision making in therapy.

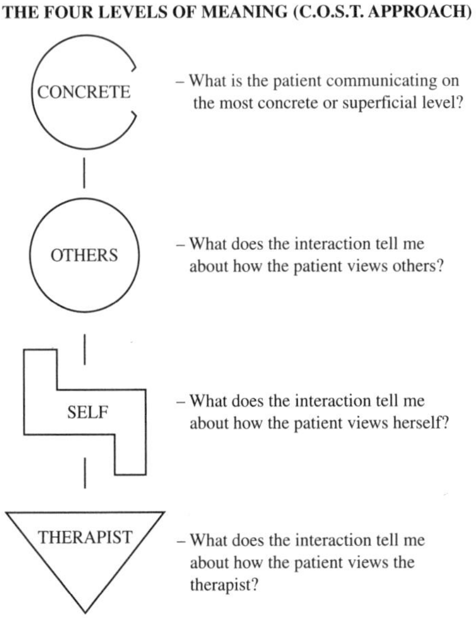
THE FOUR LEVELS OF MEANING (C.O.S.T. APPROACH)
CONCRETE
– What is the patient communicating on the most concrete or superficial level?
OTHERS
– What does the interaction tell me about how the patient views others?
SELF
– What does the interaction tell me about how the patient views herself?
THERAPIST
– What does the interaction tell me about how the patient views the therapist?

Figure 8.2 The Four Levels of Meaning (C.O.S.T Approach)

As you can see, the first letter of each of the four levels of meaning spells the acronym "C.O.S.T." As a memory aid, you can remember this as the "cost" that our patients can pay in lost or damaged relationships, as a result of untreated interpersonal problems.

1. *Concrete.* What is the patient communicating on the most concrete or superficial level? This is the level limited to the most obvious content of the person's statement or question. In this case,

Susan is talking about her new boyfriend and her concerns about this budding romantic relationship.

2. *Others.* What does the interaction tell me about how the patient views others? This can help you understand the patient's active **object representation**. In this case, Susan is describing perceiving previous boyfriends as withholding, cold, and distant, and she is wondering whether her new boyfriend will end up being just like (her perception of) the others.

3. *Self.* What does the interaction tell me about how the patient views herself? This can help you understand the patient's active **self representation**. In this case, Susan's comments suggest that she is viewing herself as a helpless, mistreated victim in her relationships.

4. *Therapist.* What does the interaction tell me about how the patient views the therapist? This also relates to the patient's active **object representation**. This part can be more difficult to piece together, particularly when the patient is not specifically—or at least not consciously—talking about the therapist. Susan has just recently begun therapy. There is a striking parallel between initiating a new romantic relationship in her personal life, and recently initiating the therapeutic relationship. It is very common for patients to unconsciously choose to discuss themes in their lives that parallel their experience of what is going on within the therapeutic relationship at the moment. We could thus speculate that it may well be Susan's uncertainty about where the *therapeutic* relationship is going that unconsciously led her to discuss her concerns about her new romantic interest. Alternatively, it is also possible that Susan's comments reflect her **object representation** of the *therapist* (who began the session with silence) as cold and distant. We could speculate that

this may have triggered memories of cold and distant relationships that she experienced in the past, leading to her comments. Sometimes it can be difficult for new therapists to accept the notion that what the patient says in therapy is so closely connected to what is going on within the therapeutic relationship, especially when the connection is not immediately obvious. Try to keep an open mind, and you may be surprised by how often this actually occurs.

In deciding what to say, the therapist can choose to address any of the four levels of meaning, from the most superficial/conscious level to the deepest (and often unconscious) ones. The therapist's choice as to which level to address can depend on many factors. Addressing the most superficial level is typically the least anxiety provoking for most patients. This can be seen as similar to a supportive style of psychotherapy. By contrast, continuously focusing only on the fourth level can be quite an intense and overwhelming experience for many patients, particularly early on during the course of therapy. I would also generally caution against choosing to address the fourth level at the very end of a session, as you may not have time to help the patient ease any resulting anxiety before the session is over.

Why might directing one's comments toward the fourth level be so intense for people? I think there are a couple of reasons for this. First, many people are quite uncomfortable with an honest, open, and direct discussion of their feelings for the person they are talking with. After all, that may be one of the reasons the patient is in therapy. As you might imagine, it can be *especially* uncomfortable talking about one's feelings for one's *therapist*. In addition, patients can be taken aback by a therapist's ability to see beyond the superficial meaning of statements, and to recognize how the seemingly unrelated themes discussed may in fact be relevant to the current therapy situation and relationship. This may be especially unsettling when the patient herself is initially unaware of a connection, and then is able to see one after it is pointed out. It is often best to gradually build up to addressing the deeper levels of meaning as the patient's capacity to tolerate a more open discussion of feelings "in the moment" develops. A reasonable rule of thumb would be to try a few times during each session to help the patient be more aware of and relate on one level deeper than the one she is currently comfortable with.

The therapist in the previous example used a somewhat ambiguous turn of phrase, "this new relationship," to simultaneously address the first and fourth levels of meaning. This leaves it open for Susan to process the statement (consciously and/or unconsciously) on either or both levels. It is helpful to be watchful for opportunities like this. In addition, notice that the therapist's statement is followed by a request that Susan describe her feelings. This reflects another important therapeutic principle in deciding what to say in therapy—that of "going after the affect." Given that the capacity to consider the four levels of meaning takes time and practice to develop, going after the affect is a useful fallback position if you are uncertain as to what to say next.

CHAPTER NINE

Tools of the Trade

In the last chapter, we discussed an approach to understanding what is occurring in the therapist–patient interaction from various perspectives. Once you have synthesized a hypothesis about what is going on, what do you actually say? And how do you say it? Do you ask a question? Do you make a statement? What are the options? In this chapter, I would like to discuss the three key types of interventions or tools of the trade used in **psychodynamic psychotherapy**, namely **clarification**, **confrontation**, and **interpretation**.

Clarification is self-explanatory. It involves any request for more information. In the last chapter, the therapist used **clarification** twice in the sample exchange with Susan. In the first instance, the therapist said: "Tell me what that's like for you." In the second instance, the therapist requested: "Tell me all about what you are feeling right now." It is clear that in both of these examples the therapist is asking for more information about something (in this case, Susan's feelings). The following are a few more examples of **clarification**: "Please go on," "I'm not sure I understand," and "Tell me all about that."

Unfortunately, **confrontation** is not quite so self-explanatory. Although the word **confrontation** sounds aggressive, this connotation is not actually pertinent to the meaning of the term as a therapeutic intervention. Just like any other intervention, **confrontation** statements or questions should be delivered with respect and courtesy. **Confrontation** involves telling the patient something about herself (i.e., *directing her attention* to it, and/or *raising awareness* of it). It may involve raising awareness of an aspect of the patient's behavior or affect state (e.g., "You seem to be enjoying being here today"). It may involve directing the patient's attention to something that she is already aware of (e.g., "I notice that you're wearing sunglasses today"). Alternatively, it may raise awareness about something that the patient is avoiding or is not consciously aware of. For example, in the previous chapter the therapist remarked: "You seem irritated, even now as you talk about it." Susan replied that she had been unaware of any feeling of irritation prior to the therapist's comment. **Confrontation** can also be helpful for raising awareness of inconsistencies. An example of this would be: "You said today that I understand you better than anyone. Just last week, however, you said that there was nothing helpful about seeing me. It seems that your view of me has switched in a pretty extreme way." Together, **clarification** and **confrontation** interventions can sometimes set up or pave the way for **interpretations**.

An **interpretation** involves a statement or question (often involving information gathered from **clarifications** and **confrontations**) that is designed to help the patient to *understand and appreciate* an internal issue or struggle that is outside of her awareness. This may involve describing a connection between what is happening in the therapeutic relationship in the here and now and past experiences (e.g., "You seem to be experiencing me today as trying to control you, much like you said your mother did when you were a child"). Alternatively, it may involve explaining why a particular affect state is being avoided. (For example: "Earlier you seemed to be experiencing positive feelings toward me. When I asked you to describe those feelings further, somehow you shifted the conversation to discussing your frustrations with work. I guess that's understandable, since you're much more familiar with feelings of irritation. Experiencing and talking about your caring feelings is less familiar and more uncomfortable for you.") **Interpretations** can also help the patient to understand and appreciate the active **object relations unit** (which consists of the relevant **self representation**, the corresponding **object representation**, and the affect experienced about the representations). For example, "You seem to be viewing me as an angry and rejecting parent, and yourself much like a fearful, hurt, and helpless child." The assumption behind making **interpretations** is that if the patient develops an appreciation and understanding of her unconscious internal conflicts (and how they manifest as interpersonal problems), it will help her to resolve them. In **object relations** therapy, **confrontations** and **interpretations** are often designed to promote integration by bringing together conflicting, disparate aspects of the patient's **self** and **object representations** that are being kept apart in the patient's mind (through the use of **splitting**[1]).

---

[1] **Splitting** is an immature **defense mechanism** that reduces anxiety by keeping notions of good and bad separate in the person's mind.

In a 4-year study by Høglend et al. (2008), it was demonstrated that 1 year of weekly **psychodynamic psychotherapy** (involving 1 to 3 **interpretations** per 45-minute session) was associated with sustained improvements on scales of psychodynamic functioning, even in patients with a lifelong pattern of severe interpersonal problems. A higher frequency of interpretations is typically not preferable, however, as this can be overwhelming for many patients. Please be aware that **interpretations** that focus on the patient's experience of the therapeutic relationship in the here and now (which are commonly used in **object relations** therapy) can be more anxiety provoking, compared to **interpretations** regarding the patient's relationships outside of therapy. For these reasons, when it comes to **interpretations**, less is often more. It is generally preferable to give more consideration to the timing and sensitive delivery of a small number of **interpretations** (perhaps even just one or two per session) than to attempt to fill the session with numerous anxiety-provoking, poorly timed **interpretations** that do not resonate with the patient.

Although I have focused on the three fundamental interventions that are most characteristic of **object relations** therapy (**clarification**, **confrontation**, and **interpretation**), it should be noted that more supportive interventions (such as **empathic validation**,[2] praise, and advice-giving) should by no means be excluded from

---

[2] **Empathic validation** involves a statement from the therapist that demonstrates attunement with the patient's emotional experience. For example: "I can understand that you would feel angry about that." **Empathic validation** can be a particularly useful technique when treating patients with prominent narcissistic traits.

your therapeutic toolkit. As with all of the suggestions and techniques discussed in this book, I would encourage you to try to select the most appropriate intervention to help the patient develop a healthier relationship with herself and others, based on a sound understanding of the situation, the patient, and her particular relationship patterns. If a particular scenario calls for supportive techniques for the attainment of the treatment goals, so be it! I think it is important not to become too attached to a specific set of interventions or techniques merely because they are the ones traditionally espoused by one's particular psychotherapeutic orientation. Although the suggestions in this text are predominantly based on an **object relations** approach, some of my suggestions reflect integration with other psychotherapy frameworks. You will find that many of the sample dialogues in the upcoming chapters demonstrate supportive interventions (especially **empathic validation**), used either on their own, or incorporated into the **clarifications**, **confrontations**, and **interpretations**.

CHAPTER TEN

Projective Identification

The concepts in this chapter are probably some of the most important to understand and apply if you are going to be performing therapy from an **object relations** perspective. So please read the chapter carefully. And once you have read it, read it again. And again. Have I convinced you that it is important? Okay let's move on.

So what is **projective identification**? **Projective identification** is a **defense mechanism** that can occur between two (or more) people. It is a concept that was coined by Melanie Klein, one of the pioneers of **object relations** psychotherapy, in 1946. Essentially, it involves the following two steps:

1. One person (e.g., the patient) behaves in a way that projects an intolerable thought or emotion onto another person (e.g., the therapist). This is the **projection** part of the process.

2. The recipient (e.g., the therapist) begins to feel and behave as if characterized by this thought or emotion. This is the **identification** part of the process.

This **defense mechanism** serves to unconsciously rid the patient of unacceptable feelings or beliefs by projecting them onto the recipient. Pathological **projective identification** and **splitting** are two hallmark **defense mechanisms** of the borderline personality. However, these **defense mechanisms** can also occur in those with predominantly healthy relationships. Indeed, I would suggest to you that some form of **projective identification** is going on most of the time in all relationships, and this is not necessarily pathological.

Unfortunately, recognizing pathological **projective identification** in therapy is not always a simple matter. Even the most seasoned therapist can miss it. It requires constant vigilance over one's emotional reaction to what is going on. This is because **projective identification** involves tremendous pressure for the recipient to *unconsciously* identify with the projection. In addition, pathological **projective identification** often involves a projected sense of urgency: "Fix it now! Do something now! React now!" Recognizing this feeling of urgency when talking with a patient is a fairly sensitive tip-off that **projective identification** may be at work in some way. Let's consider an example of this process in action.

(Susan was 20 minutes late for her appointment last week. When she arrived, she initially stated that she had been late because she had missed her bus. Instead of accepting this answer at face value, the therapist enquired further about the events that had led Susan to miss her bus. Susan told the therapist that she had left work and gone home for lunch before her therapy appointment. Prior to leaving home to catch her bus, Susan had phoned a friend to discuss the possibility of getting together on the weekend. Susan acknowledged that the possibility of missing her bus had occurred to her during her rather lengthy telephone conversation. She stated that the phone chat somehow seemed "more important than being on time for therapy." She went on to say that even though she wanted and valued therapy, the prospect of arriving late to her therapy session "didn't seem like a big deal at the time." This led to a discussion of Susan's discomfort with acknowledging and tolerating her need for therapy. Despite this discussion at last week's appointment, Susan arrives 12 minutes late for today's session. She finds the door open and she walks in with a smile as she greets the therapist.)

Susan: "Hi! How are you today?"

Therapist: "I'm well, thanks. Please have a seat."

Susan: "Well, I've had an interesting week. Jane, the other receptionist at the office, was fired this week . . . " (Susan goes on to describe the events at her office leading to her co-worker being fired. This description goes on for approximately 5 minutes, leading to a natural pause.)

Therapist: "I notice that you were late arriving again this week, Susan." (**confrontation**)

Susan: "Oh yeah, I just had to take care of a few last-minute things before leaving home, and I guess I lost track of the time. My bad!"

> Therapist: "I'm concerned about how coming late for your appointments could affect your therapy. Can you help me understand in more detail what seems to be happening that's leading you to arrive after your appointment has already begun?" (**clarification**)
>
> Susan: "I was only a few minutes late, what's the big deal? Are you paid by the minute or something?"

If you were to put yourself in the place of the therapist in the example above, how do you imagine you would feel in response to Susan's last comment? She is implying that you are overreacting. This comment reflects an attack on your neediness as a therapist ("*You* need me to be on time . . . *You* are overreacting"). Susan is also implying that your response to her tardiness is rooted in financial self-concern, rather than true concern for her well-being. It is not hard to see that a therapist might feel irritated by such comments and their implications. So the main feeling that Susan is projecting onto the therapist appears to be anger. We could hypothesize that Susan is feeling angry as a reaction to intolerance of her need for therapy, which likely led to her lateness in the first place. Here is where the fork in the road occurs for the therapist. Do you, as the therapist, recognize in this moment that the irritation you are feeling (or being induced to feel) reflects projected feelings from the patient? Or do you unconsciously identify with those feelings as your own, and become overtly irritated at Susan? A therapist's ability to analyze what is happening and choose a *therapeutic* (rather than reflexive) response/course of action is a key feature that distinguishes the therapeutic relationship from other relationships in our patients' lives. This therapeutic response to pathological **projective identification** can give the patient the opportunity to "take back" what is being projected (in this case

Susan's anger regarding her need for therapy), but in a new, metabolized form—after the therapist has processed it and chosen a therapeutic way/form to return it to the patient.

So to return to our example, how might you respond in the above situation? Hopefully, you are now considering the four levels of meaning (C.O.S.T.) covered in Chapter Eight (The Four Levels of Meaning). It would be a useful exercise at this point to jot down some thoughts about the dialogue above, and how to understand it according to each of the four levels. On the most superficial/concrete level, Susan is angry at you for your supposed neediness, greediness, and overreaction. On the second level, we could speculate that Susan may tend to react with anger to perceived neediness in others. What do her comments and emotional reaction tell us about her relationship with herself? It seems likely—particularly given the discussion during the previous session—that Susan is intolerant of her feelings of neediness. This is a very common problem.

How might we understand what is going on in her relationship with the therapist? This is where things can get a little bit tricky. As mentioned above, we have hypothesized that Susan is intolerant of her need for others. This could create a state of intrapsychic conflict and tension within her. On the one hand, she seems to recognize that she wants and needs therapy. On the other hand, she feels irritated by the feelings of neediness that therapy stirs up within her. In an unconscious effort to rid herself of the consequent tension, she behaves in a way that creates a similar conflict between you and her (by arriving late), projecting her intolerable feelings (i.e., her feelings of yearning and need) onto you. She then perceives *you* as the needy one in the relationship (because of your stated need for her to be on time) and attacks the neediness that she now perceives in you. You have become the owner of all of that distasteful neediness. She no longer perceives it as originating from within herself. This has effectively taken a conflict that was initially going on within her mind (i.e., Susan attacking *her own* neediness) and created a seemingly external conflict—in which she is attacking the neediness she now perceives in you. Can you see how that might provide relief for her? The conflict that initially resided solely within her mind is now perceived to be between you and her, and *you* are viewed as the one responsible for it—because you are behaving in such a pathetically needy way. In addition, most of this—apart perhaps from her irritation at you—is occurring outside of Susan's conscious awareness.

If one were to put all this together in terms of an activated **object relations unit**, Susan appears to be experiencing anger (the affect) in response to viewing herself as mistreated and attacked (the **self representation**) by a needy, greedy, overreacting therapist (the **object representation**). Hopefully, I have explained all of this in a way that makes sense to you. It can take a while sometimes to wrap your mind around these concepts. This is well worth doing, however, as it is from this understanding that we can develop and weigh options for how to proceed.

Now that we have reviewed our understanding of the situation using the four levels of meaning, the next thing to do is to decide which level to gear a response to. Given that Susan is directly addressing an issue between her and you, I think it makes sense to formulate a response tailored to the fourth level of meaning. Remember, her last question to you was: "I was only a few minutes late, what's the big deal? Are you paid by the minute or something?"

Let's consider a few response options. I will typically consider three "intensities" of response: essentially gentle, moderate, and intense. A gentle response typically does not address the relationship between patient and therapist. In that way is it is more of a "supportive" response or comment. A moderate-intensity response would indirectly address what is going on in the therapeutic relationship. And an intense response would involve directly addressing what is going on within the therapeutic relationship (i.e., addressing **transference**[1] issues). A fairly gentle response to the above situation might be the following: "You seem frustrated. (**confrontation**) Why don't you tell me all about how you're feeling right now?" (**clarification**) A moderate-intensity response might be: "You seem quite irritated *with me*. (**confrontation**) Perhaps you can tell me what's going on for you right now?" (**clarification**) An intense response might be: "My expectation that you are here on time must seem pathetic and irritating. (**confrontation**) What's it like for you to see me as so demanding?" (**clarification**) Notice that each of these responses invites Susan to describe her affect state further.

The above responses are all essentially directed at Susan's irritation at the therapist's neediness. How patients tolerate and respond to their neediness (and perceived neediness in others) tends to be a prominent and recurring theme in therapy. The therapist could instead have chosen to focus on Susan's implication that the therapist is only interested in her punctuality because of greediness. Can you think of some ways to address this issue? (Hint: notice that in the example responses above, the therapist does not defend against Susan's misguided implications, but rather rolls with the implications of the attack, e.g., "What's it like for you to see me as so demanding?")

---

[1] **Transference** is the process by which a patient unconsciously and inaccurately perceives the therapist as possessing qualities that characterized important figures from her past (often a parent).

CHAPTER ELEVEN

Anxiety and the Paranoid-Schizoid Position

The concept of the **paranoid-schizoid position** can be a confusing one for therapists who are new to **object relations**. It is a useful concept to understand, however, as many of our patients spend much of their time in this state. The term was initially coined by Melanie Klein (1946) to describe the infantile state of panic and terror that occurs when a baby's needs are not being met. The infant perceives the situation as an attack on its life. When trying to understand the **paranoid-schizoid position**, it is helpful to break the term down into its constituent components. The "paranoid" component refers to anxiety and terror regarding perceived persecution or attack from the outside world. The "schizoid" part refers to the split between "all good" (i.e., goodness within the individual) and "all bad" (i.e., malevolence emanating from the outside world).

Can you recall ever being in a situation that you felt was catastrophic and overwhelming? Do you remember the anxiety and panic you felt at the time? We can all enter this frame of mind from time to time, given the right set of circumstances. Can you imagine how it would feel to be in this "red-alert, catastrophic meltdown" state *most* of the time? This is the case for many individuals suffering with severe interpersonal pathology. Almost any situation or interaction can be perceived as a threat to their very existence. Perhaps you can imagine how emotionally draining that could get, day after day. This is one reason why helping our patients to develop the capacity to regulate their anxiety and distress is so important.

In an earlier section we talked about how to help our patients become better observers of their emotions, rather than being carried away and overwhelmed by them. One way to accomplish this is by engaging the patient in describing her emotional state in as much detail as possible. Describing an emotional state verbally can be challenging for many patients, and I will often tell patients so for reassurance, if they are having difficulty with this. As I had stated earlier, most patients find it easiest to start by describing how their emotions are affecting them *physically*. You can then ask the patient to describe her *thoughts* about the situation in detail. Lastly, the patient can describe what the emotion itself is like in more *abstract* terms (perhaps using metaphors or similes, e.g., "It's like I'm in a dark room and I can't see what's going on." The importance of practicing and developing this capacity cannot be overstated. It is perhaps why psychotherapists have become known for the famous therapy question: How does that make you feel? The following is an example of how to help the patient engage in this process.

Susan: "Can you believe she said that to me? What if my boss was there, what would *he* think?"

Therapist: "That does sound like it was stressful for you. I can see that you're feeling quite tense right now, just talking about it." (**confrontation**)

Susan: "Well, yeah, wouldn't you? What if she starts saying things like that to other people at work? I wouldn't be surprised if I lost my job!"

Therapist: "Susan, describe to me what you're feeling right now." (**clarification**)

Susan: "What am I *feeling*? I'm feeling like she's trying to get me fired!"

Therapist: "You certainly seem pretty tense. (**confrontation**) Can you tell me where you're feeling that tension in your body?" (**clarification**)

Susan: "I'm feeling tense everywhere! It feels like my stomach is tied in knots."

Therapist: "I see. Where else are you feeling the tension?" (**clarification**)

Susan: "Well, my leg muscles feel tight . . . and so does my neck and back."

Therapist: "What else do you notice about that tension physically?" (**clarification**)

Susan: "My hands are gripping the arms of the chair."

Therapist: "What's going through your mind right now?" (**clarification**)

Susan: "I can't believe this keeps happening to me. It is *so* frustrating."

Therapist: "I can understand that you would feel pretty frustrated about what she said. Tell me about the frustration you feel. Describe it to me in as much detail as possible." (**clarification**)

Susan: "It's like I just start to see red . . . the whole world starts to close in around me. I start to worry, and then things just seem to mushroom out of control . . . I'm feeling a little calmer now, though."

Therapist: "You *do* seem calmer now. (**confrontation**) When you're able to observe your feelings in detail like we do here, it seems to help." (**confrontation**)

Susan: "Yeah, it does help when you take me through it, but what about when you're not around?"

Can you piece together Susan's activated **object relations unit** in the dialogue above? How is she experiencing herself? How is she viewing her co-worker? What is the affect linking the two views? Susan seems to perceive herself as the innocent victim of a malevolent co-worker who is bent on destroying her. Susan's affect seems terrified and infuriated, reminiscent of a fight-or-flight reaction.

The therapist was able to help Susan engage in the act of observing her emotional state. This can be challenging at times when the patient is in the throes of the **paranoid-schizoid position**. Sometimes patients will begin to describe their feelings, only to veer off topic and start to spin out of control again. If this keeps happening over and over, you can comment on it to the patient: "I notice that when I ask you to describe your feelings, you begin to do so, but then you switch to talking about something else." (**confrontation**) Sometimes a comment like this is enough to help the patient refocus, rather than be swept away by intense emotion. You may need to refocus the patient like this a few times, however. This process can help patients to develop conscious awareness of the shifts in their mental state. This can also develop into an even more collaborative process in which the patient may begin to identify these shifts on her own: "Oh, I think I just did it again!"

Notice that at the end of the dialogue, Susan asked about how she can cope when the therapist is not there to help. During the session, Susan is able to make use of the therapist's calming presence and guidance to calm herself down. Why is this more difficult between appointments, when Susan is alone? In part, this may reflect a poorly developed capacity for **object constancy**, mentioned in Chapter Four (Assessment and Formulation). Remember, this involves the capacity to maintain a stable and accurate mental representation of a person in his or her absence. Between appointments, Susan may hold a primarily negative view of the therapist— experiencing him or her as rejecting and abandoning. She may find it difficult to access and make use of a calming mental representation of the therapist when he or she is not physically present. Thus, between sessions Susan finds it even more difficult than usual to view the therapist in a balanced way that reflects coexisting frustrating and satisfying qualities. It is important to try to help our patients to develop this capacity.

So what can we do to help foster **object constancy** in our patients? In the example given above, the therapist might suggest that Susan could try imagining being in therapy when she is feeling distressed between appointments. I often advocate trying this for the first time when the patient is somewhere where she will not be disturbed (e.g., alone at home). It is usually too difficult to try this for the first time when one is in the midst of a stressful situation in public. I might suggest that Susan sit down in her home and describe (either mentally, out loud, or in writing) her emotional state in detail (while imagining hearing my voice guiding her through it—just like during her sessions with me). Susan can also reflect on her thoughts and feelings about the therapist as a part of this process. Practicing this can help develop **object constancy** by helping Susan to access a positive, calming representation of the therapist, instead of focusing solely on a negative representation and associated affect. Of course, the primary way that **object constancy** will develop is through the consistency of therapy itself, along with repeated exploration of the changes in the patient's experience of the therapist.

Patients who are lacking **object constancy** and who have a tendency toward the **paranoid-schizoid position** often respond well to reassurance about the future—that is, that there *is* one for them. Remember, the **paranoid-schizoid position** involves an exaggerated fear of persecution and annihilation. Once you have helped the person to calm down adequately, she can then hear and make use of reassuring comments that can help strengthen aspects of **object constancy**. The following are examples of such reassuring comments: "We have lots of time ahead of us, both today and in the coming weeks, to go over this in as much detail as you would like," and "You've been through difficult situations like this before, and you've come through them every time." Can you see how such comments could be reassuring for people? They emphasize the fact that it is not "now or never, do or die, all-or-nothing." Not only will the patient get through this situation, but you will also be there, week after week to help her through it.

CHAPTER TWELVE

Silence and Boredom in Therapy

We have already talked about how we would prefer to avoid imposing our own agenda on the therapy session. We have also discussed letting patients begin talking whenever they are ready, at the beginning of the session. If we are not leading the session with questions and topics, it follows that there may be periods of silence. These pauses can feel awkward at first, both for the patient and for the beginning therapist. With time, you will feel more comfortable with silence and you will become less focused on your own anxiety in such situations. This will free you up to focus on the patient's affect during the pauses. Silence can be connected with virtually any type of affect, depending on the context in which it is occurring. So even when there is nothing being said during a session, it is important to remain observant of the emotional tone in the room. It is very unusual for a patient to remain silent for an entire session (or even a series of sessions), though I have seen this in rare instances with individuals who struggled with quite severe interpersonal pathology.

Why am I suggesting that we avoid initiating the discussion in the therapy session? I mentioned above that we typically do not want to impose our own agenda on the session. Why would that be? It allows us to more clearly see the issues that the patient is bringing to the session without contaminating this with our own needs, interests, or feelings. In that way, whatever occurs in the session, and whatever emotional reaction you experience, you can be more certain that these reflect issues and emotions that the patient is introducing. This reflects an important therapeutic assumption that is related to **projective identification**: that your emotional reactions in the session typically reflect the patient's experience and its impact on you in the moment. That is, if I experience an emotional reaction to what is going on in therapy, I will typically assume that the shift in my affect state (or my appreciation of interpersonal pressure designed to induce such a shift) is related to what is going on for the patient in the room (reflecting **projective identification**). Thus, if I am feeling caring feelings for the patient, I will seek to understand what may have happened to cause the patient to experience stronger caring feelings for me. Likewise, if I feel emotionally nudged toward irritation, anxiety, confusion, or erotic interest. You may wonder if this is too big an assumption to make. I would contend that it is important that we make this assumption in order to be effective as psychodynamic therapists. I would go even further by stating that most of my work in therapy rests upon this assumption. Otherwise, I would constantly be second-guessing my understanding of what is going on. That is not to say that we should turn a blind eye to issues that we as therapists may be bringing to the session. If I am already overwhelmed by a personal issue outside of therapy, or if I am feeling a particularly strong emotion prior to the start of the session, then this could clearly influence my perspective and judgment. This would be another example of **negative countertransference**. This issue highlights the importance of entering each session with a "neutral emotional palette"— to avoid creating a biased filter through which one views what is happening. Clearly, it is also important to address any significant issues in one's life (i.e., potential **negative countertransference** issues) that could interfere with one's ability to clearly see what is going on in therapy.

There are often particular "trigger issues" within the therapist's life that can contaminate therapy. These may range from strong reactivity or rigidity regarding one's opinion about certain life issues (e.g., politics, abortion, religion) to a history of some sort of abuse. When these trigger issues are discussed in therapy, it is as if the therapist suddenly puts on opaque glasses and everything seems dark and foggy through them. He or she may lose objectivity, perspective, and judgment. We all have our own set of trigger issues, and it is very important to try to be aware of them and their possible negative impact on our patients. The upshot of this is that if you know you have a trigger issue (or two, or ten), it behooves you to address this (e.g., through your own therapy), and be sure to explore how it may have influenced the session during your psychotherapy supervision.

Coming back to the issue of silence in therapy, sometimes patients will wonder if sitting in silence during therapy is a waste of time. Questions about this can reflect a number of affect states, ranging from interested concern to overt anger. Thus, as always, you will want to consider the context when formulating your response to questions about this. I will often reassure patients that sitting together in silence *is* in fact doing something useful. The patient might say that she could just as easily be sitting at home alone, not talking. This is not the case, however. The patient is sitting in a room, in silence, with *you*. This is an entirely different experience than sitting at home alone. Learning to tolerate silence in relationships is an important skill in and of itself. In addition, periods of silence in therapy are often connected with a significant amount of affect. I will typically focus my attention on uncovering the affect arising out of silences (and/or the affect that led to the silence in the first place). In addition, I will use the time to think about how to understand the silence using the C.O.S.T. approach. It would be somewhat unusual, however, for me to be the one to break the silence. I would typically prefer to see where it goes, and let the patient speak, when and if she is ready. If the periods of silence are prolonged and repeated over multiple sessions, this would typically constitute significant **resistance**[1] to therapeutic progress. Understanding the context and patterns that develop, perhaps even over a number of sessions, may eventually shed light on the meaning and significance of the silence.

The development of boredom in a therapy session is always significant. People sometimes conceptualize boredom as the absence of emotion. I would argue that this is not the case. Rather, boredom can be thought of as "crushing of emotion." This is an active and effortful process. Why else would boredom feel so draining? If I find myself feeling bored in a therapy session, I will consider what is going on in the relationship

---

[1] **Resistance** can be defined as the patient's conscious and/or unconscious opposition to the treatment.

(i.e., via **projective identification**) and review what this tells me about the patient's experience. I will pay particular attention to my emotional reactions to the patient (in addition to considering the "hear" and "observe" parts of the H.O.R.S.E. approach) to try to uncover what emotions the patient may be avoiding or "crushing." I will then try to understand what this means according to the four levels of meaning (i.e., the C.O.S.T. approach). These steps typically help me understand the important themes that relate to boredom in the moment.

People often consciously or unconsciously blame boredom on their environment (e.g., a boring lecturer, television show, or novel). This commonly leads to feelings of irritation (e.g., with the therapist). So irritation is often the affect state that will need to be addressed on one of the four levels of meaning we discussed earlier. (Have you noticed that irritation with the therapist seems to come up a fair bit?) The following is an example of a dialogue that might occur related to this issue:

Therapist: "You seem a little drained as you talk to me today." (**confrontation**) (Including "me" in the question may help the patient talk about her feelings within the context of the therapeutic relationship, rather than just talking about her feelings as if they exist in a vacuum.)

Susan: "Yeah, I guess. I feel like I'm always the one talking, telling you all about my life, and you just sit there and listen and don't say anything about your life at all. I don't know the first thing about you." (She says with a clearly irritated tone.)

Therapist: "I see. There *is* an imbalance in this relationship. I imagine you find that quite irritating." (**confrontation**)

Susan: "Like you said, it's not balanced."
Therapist: "Tell me all about the irritation you are feeling."
  (**clarification**)

What is Susan communicating about the relationship with the therapist (i.e., the "T" in C.O.S.T.) in the dialogue above? Susan is describing her perception that the therapeutic relationship is too "one-sided." Her comments convey anger at the therapist, whom she appears to be viewing as a rejecting and withholding authority figure—the relevant **object representation**. It makes sense, then, that the therapist comments on her irritation and explores this further.

Another option in this situation would be to focus on Susan's developing curiosity about the therapist. This developing interest reflects her growing desire for attachment. But where is the affect related to this yearning for attachment? It seems to be obscured and overshadowed by Susan's anger. It is quite possible that Susan is unaware of the underlying desire for attachment suggested by her comments. Her anger could be viewed as "defending against" her desire for attachment—a desire that can initially be overwhelming to think and talk about for many patients.[2] One might therefore expect that focusing on Susan's growing curiosity about the thera-pist might constitute a more intense and anxiety-provoking

---

[2] This can be viewed as a superficial "angry" **object relations unit** defending against an underlying and overwhelming "yearning for attach-ment" **object relations unit**. Can you piece together the relevant **self** and **object representations**?

intervention in this situation. The following is an example of how that conversation might go:

> Therapist: "You seem a little drained as you talk to me today." (**confrontation**)
>
> Susan: "Yeah, I guess. I feel like I'm always the one talking, telling you all about my life, and you just sit there and listen and don't say anything about your life at all. I don't know the first thing about you." (She says with a clearly irritated tone.)
>
> Therapist: "I see. There *is* an imbalance in this relationship. I would imagine that might be irritating for you. But I wonder if there is more to it than that. I wonder if in part you are also telling me that you are developing some curiosity about me and my personal life?" (**confrontation**)
>
> Susan: "Well, maybe . . . but then again, I'm not sure I want to know too much about you."
>
> Therapist: "You sort of do, but you also sort of don't?" (**clarification**)
>
> Susan: "That's right." (Readjusts her seating position.)
>
> Therapist: "Well, you've been coming here for a number of weeks now, and we've been talking about your life and your feelings in a way that I suspect is unlike other relationships that you've had. I think it's pretty normal to have some feelings about that, and those feelings can be pretty strong sometimes. You agreed a moment ago that you felt drained. I wonder if you were feeling drained as a way of avoiding feeling uncomfortable or even annoyed about your curiosity about me, particularly given the

imbalances in this relationship that you just pointed out."
(**interpretation**)

Susan: "Maybe . . . I think I *was* kind of feeling irritated. It's actually kind of weird to think that I might be interested in knowing more about my therapist . . . it's all a little confusing." (Fidgets in her seat and appears somewhat anxious.)

Therapist: "It *is* a little confusing. As I said, I think the curiosity you are experiencing is pretty normal. I can understand that it's not an easy thing for you to talk about. You seem a bit uneasy. (**confrontation**) Tell me about how you're feeling right now." (**clarification**) (Susan goes on to describe her anxiety in detail and begins to feel more settled within a few minutes.)

You can see that this path was more anxiety provoking for Susan. That is likely because talking about anger/frustration is much more commonplace and familiar for most people, compared to discussing one's growing feelings of attachment. The latter can be much more anxiety provoking. It is often tempting for therapists to choose the path of least resistance by repeatedly focusing on the patient's anger and ignoring her underlying positive feelings. Being aware of this temptation may help you avoid this pitfall. One way to think of it (and I have often used variations of this explanation when discussing this with patients) is that many of our patients are already experts about more negative feelings like anger or self-criticism. I would argue that they probably do not need extra help with those emotions nearly as much as with experiencing and talking about more positive, caring/loving feelings.

Patients need our guidance and help with forming and maintaining mature, caring relationships. A big part of this involves developing comfort with talking about one's caring feelings *with* the person we care about. Early on, patients will often focus more on negative feelings, partly because they so often dominate their emotional state. As underlying feelings of attachment develop, most patients will increasingly introduce their particular style of relationship pathology into the sessions. Whatever seems to go wrong in their other relationships will also increasingly affect the therapeutic relationship as the feelings of attachment grow stronger. This is a normal and expected development in therapy. It is an important reason why we need not dictate what is discussed—the issues will always present themselves anyway.[3] As patients move forward in therapy and develop tolerance of their own neediness, they are able to focus more and more on experiencing and describing their caring feelings. This typically progresses from discussing and describing caring feelings regarding relationships outside of therapy (which is easier), to developing comfort with discussing caring feelings in the context of the therapeutic relationship (i.e., focusing more on the fourth level of meaning). When a patient is able to do so in a forthright and healthy manner, without experiencing overwhelming anxiety, and without introducing a pathological style of interaction (e.g., **idealization** of the

---

[3] This relates to a fundamental psychodynamic concept called **psychic determinism**. According to this concept, a person's behavior and intrapsychic processes are never viewed as random or coincidental, but rather as inextricably linked to unconscious forces that exist as a result of past experiences.

therapist, or use of pathological **projective identification**), I typically view this as a strong indicator of progress. It follows that an important therapeutic goal should involve helping patients to shift from focusing on predominantly negative (e.g., frustration/anger, self-loathing) to predominantly positive affects states (e.g., feelings of affection/caring). Furthermore, it is important to gradually help our patients develop comfort discussing these feelings in the moment, with the person (i.e., the therapist) they are having feelings about. Once the patient is able to have a mature, caring relationship with the therapist that is open, direct, honest, and respectful of therapeutic relationship boundaries, then the patient has very likely developed the capacity to do so in other relationships as well.

I would suggest, however, that the shift to helping the patient focus on her more positive feelings needs to occur gradually and according to the patient's capacity to tolerate and articulate strong caring emotions. Adapting to each patient's particular pace is a skill you will have to develop over time. Press the issue and the patient may become overwhelmed and overly anxious. She may even decompensate or drop out of therapy altogether as a result. Move too slowly and therapy can stagnate or become entrenched in a habitual negative focus.

Because focusing on positive, caring feelings often increases anxiety, you must be prepared to help your patient settle in these situations. And that may take some time in the session. As you might expect, it is often ill advised to focus on such anxiety-provoking material at the very end of the appointment.

CHAPTER THIRTEEN

Neediness in Therapy

You may recall that I have referred to neediness in discussing some of the examples in previous chapters. Understanding and addressing how our patients deal with neediness in relationships is a very important part of **object relations** therapy. Most of the patients I have worked with have had significant difficulties tolerating their neediness in relationships. This issue seems to come up again and again in various ways. If someone is unable to tolerate needing another person, how can she possibly tolerate having a relationship? Needing others in itself is not usually the problem. All mature, loving relationships involve feelings of neediness. Problems tend to arise when people are unable to *tolerate* the vulnerability and intensity of emotion that is involved. It is thus very important to help our patients learn to tolerate both the depth of their own neediness, as well as their perception of neediness in others.

We discussed neediness when reviewing a dialogue between Susan and her therapist in Chapter Ten (Projective Identification). If you will recall, Susan became angry when the therapist commented on her tardiness. We discussed her neediness with regard to the second through fourth levels of meaning. This example illustrated that Susan's reaction to neediness was to attack it. This is a very common reaction. If one considers how this tendency might arise developmentally, perhaps it makes sense that a child might tend to despise or disavow her neediness rather than despise her caregiver (on whom she depends for her very survival) for not meeting her needs to her satisfaction.

It is important to be aware of neediness in the therapeutic relationship and to observe how our patients respond to neediness within themselves, as well as expressions of neediness from others. Ask yourself: Who does the patient perceive as the needy one in the relationship right now? How is she reacting to this? Does she tend to attack neediness? Is she consciously aware of her neediness? Or is it so overwhelming that it is kept outside of her conscious awareness? The manner and intensity with which a patient reacts to neediness reflects the degree of interpersonal pathology she is prone to.

So what do you do once you notice the patient experiencing difficulties tolerating neediness in the therapeutic relationship? I would suggest that you use the H.O.R.S.E. approach (remembering to pay particular attention to your emotional reaction to the patient) to uncover what the patient is communicating about her reaction to neediness; formulate an understanding of this (using the C.O.S.T. approach); and use **confrontation** and/or **interpretation** to promote conscious awareness of her difficulties with experiencing neediness in relationships.

While you are developing experience with sorting this out, addressing the patient's affect state remains, as always, a useful interim measure. After the session, I would suggest breaking the situation down further (preferably with your psychotherapy supervisor) so that you can think about the situation from various perspectives and consider the different options that were available to you. After reviewing situations like this many, many times, you will begin to better understand what is happening *during* the session itself. Once that happens, you will then begin to see your options more clearly in the heat of the moment. Let's look at another example of neediness in a dialogue with Susan so that we can practice breaking the situation down:

> Susan: "I'm not sure how this is supposed to be helping me. I don't know what you want me to talk about. I can't really see where this is going. Can you tell me how this is supposed to be helping me?" (She asks with an irritated tone.)
>
> Therapist: "You sound irritated. And you are describing uncertainty about where therapy is going. (**confrontation**) Before I try to answer your question, it would help me to understand more about what's going on for you, and what is behind your concerns. Please tell me all about it." (**clarification**)
>
> Susan: "Well, I come here week after week and I don't even know what I'm supposed to talk about. You don't really say much or tell me what I should be working on. If this is just about me coming here and talking about anything, I could do that with my friends."

Therapist: "I see. So coming here and talking to me feels just like when you talk with your friends?" (**clarification**)

Susan: "Yes . . . well, no, not really—I guess it *is* kind of different."

Therapist: "How would you say it's different?" (**clarification**)

Susan: "Well, when I talk with my friends, they talk about their lives too. You don't say too much. Well that's not true, you *do* talk. But it's different than with my friends. Here we usually end up talking about my feelings."

Therapist: "I see. I guess in a way you've answered your question about where therapy is going. You've already noticed that therapy seems to be moving towards your feelings. And it's not easy to talk about your feelings, especially while you are experiencing them." (**confrontation**)

Susan: "No, it's not. It's kind of intense sometimes. But I think it would be nice to be able to talk about feelings in my normal relationships too."

Let's try to go through the dialogue above. Susan is asking a rather pointed question of the therapist, putting him or her on the spot. This can be seen as fairly aggressive on her part. She appears to be projecting her feelings of discomfort, urgency, and frustration. The therapist comments on Susan's irritation and paraphrases the theme of uncertainty in therapy, implying a possible connection with her feelings of irritability. Notice that the therapist chose not to answer her question right away, but rather asked for **clarification**. The therapist did not reflexively respond to the projected urgency to "Give me the answer now!" before taking the time to better understand the situation. Susan then comments on her perception that there is a lack of guidance from the therapist as to what she should talk about in therapy. This might well be triggering anxiety and irritation due to Susan's feelings of neediness—for the guidance that she perceives the therapist to be withholding. Susan attacks therapy (and the therapist) by suggesting that it is no different than talking with her friends. Her anger links the same **self** and **object representations** we discussed in the previous chapter—that is, perceiving herself as the neglected victim of a distant and withholding authority figure. The therapist's **clarification** questions lead Susan to consider the inaccuracy of these **self** and **object representations**. She identifies a distinction between her relationship with the therapist and her friendships. She begins to realize that the therapist is very attentive to her feelings. This is at once overwhelming and desirable to her, as evidenced by her comment about how nice it would be to be able to talk about her feelings in her other relationships. The therapist then focuses on the third level of meaning (i.e., the "S" in C.O.S.T.). He or she provides reassurance (via **confrontation**) about how difficult it is for Susan to talk about her feelings in the moment. This comment, which recognizes her struggle, would likely promote a deepening of therapeutic rapport.[1]

When thinking about the dialogue as a whole, Susan appears to be upset about her perception of a lack of guidance from the therapist. She seems to want the therapist to "give more" and disclose more in the sessions. This desire reflects her growing feelings of attachment and a wish for emotional reciprocity.

---

[1] This is an example of how **confrontation** can be used to convey empathy.

She may sense that her growing feelings for the therapist are stronger than the therapist's feelings for her—which is likely an accurate perception. Susan's experience of neediness results from a combination of her growing feelings of attachment and her tendency to experience the therapist as distant and withholding. If the therapist were to focus more explicitly on the fourth level of meaning (the relationship between patient and therapist) in the exchange, he or she might discuss the following: *(1)* Susan's superficial angry reaction to the imbalances in the relationship, *(2)* her underlying desire for attachment with the therapist, or *(3)* both of the above. These would all involve a more intense and direct discussion of what is taking place within the therapeutic relationship. Let's pick up part of the way through the dialogue and see where focusing on the first of these three options might have led:

> Susan: "Well, I come here week after week and I don't even know what I'm supposed to talk about. You don't really say much or tell me what I should be working on. If this is just about me coming here and talking about anything, I could do that with my friends."
>
> Therapist: "You seem to be experiencing me as distant and withholding, much like you described your father treating you when you were a child. I would imagine that might leave you feeling quite alone in this relationship, so I guess I can understand the irritation you seem to be feeling towards me." (**interpretation**)
>
> Susan: "It is kind of irritating. I don't even know anything about you. And I have no idea at all what you are writing about me."

87

Therapist: "It sounds like part of you would like to know what I think about you." (**confrontation**)

Susan: "Yes... well... I wouldn't mind reading your notes."

Therapist: "You'd like to know what I think about you but you'd prefer to find out by reading my notes, rather than by talking about it directly with me. (**confrontation**) I guess I can understand that—talking about it directly would likely involve more intense feelings." (**interpretation**)

Susan: (Silent, appears somewhat anxious.)

In this version of the dialogue, Susan's expression of neediness in the therapeutic relationship led the therapist to use an **interpretation** (combined with **empathic validation**) to identify Susan's **object representation** (i.e., her view of the therapist as distant and withholding) and suggest a connection with her irritated affect state. Can you see how according to the fourth level of meaning, Susan's request to read the therapist's process notes can be viewed as a way for her to learn about the therapist's thoughts and feelings about her *without* having to engage in open discussion about them? The therapist's **interpretation** of this may well have triggered a more conscious awareness of the intensity of her growing attachment. This could understandably have led to the anxiety and discomfort that Susan displayed thereafter, as feelings of attachment are often experienced as anxiety provoking and overwhelming. We could speculate that the discomfort she was experiencing was likely related to her realization that her therapist could "see" her growing feelings of attachment. At that point, the therapist could have asked Susan to describe her affect state in detail, with a view to helping her soothe her anxiety and develop tolerance for her caring feelings. If Susan had accepted the therapist's **interpretation** about her intense feelings without undue anxiety, he or she may then have invited Susan to further describe her feelings of attachment and desire to be cared for by the therapist. Perhaps you noticed that, just as in the last chapter, Susan's more superficial, angry feelings seemed to "cover up" or defend against her underlying desire for attachment with the therapist. Can you think of an **interpretation** that illustrates and explains this?

I hope it is evident from the discussion above that there is a connection between neediness and loving/caring feelings. Some patients respond to neediness with anger, others with anxiety. The distress can be so intense that the patient may employ **defense mechanisms** to keep the experience of neediness outside of conscious awareness. I often mention to patients that the depth of one's neediness in relationships is reflective of one's capacity to experience loving/caring feelings. Likewise, attacking or avoiding one's neediness can be viewed as attacking or avoiding one's capacity for loving feelings. If we can help our patients to better tolerate and accept the depth of their neediness and vulnerability, we can help them to overcome a common obstacle to creating healthier, more fulfilling relationships.

CHAPTER FOURTEEN

Addressing Possible Decompensation

Decompensation can be defined as any deterioration in the patient's functioning. The patient's functioning may decompensate within therapy, outside of therapy, or in both spheres. Decompensation can occur for a variety of reasons and can therefore present in various ways. It may be caused by an issue that is related to therapy itself, external life issues (e.g., medical illness, overwhelming stress due to job loss, a death in the family), or both. The patient may begin or escalate use of immature, unhealthy **defense mechanisms** that can sabotage therapy. She may develop problematic anxiety symptoms, depressive symptoms, or psychotic symptoms, which may necessitate modification or termination of her existing psychotherapy treatment. In the following example, the therapist is exploring whether Susan may be developing a depressive episode:

(Susan sits down to begin her appointment. She remains silent for approximately 30 seconds before speaking . . .)

Susan: "Well, this week was just terrible."

Therapist: (Remains silent.)

Susan: "I've been feeling really drained all week. I haven't been going out much because I've felt so out of it. I told Jeff that I didn't feel like getting together last night."

Therapist: "That does sound like a difficult week. Tell me all about it." (The therapist wonders whether this combination of a "terrible week," fatigue, and possible decreased interest might be suggestive of an evolving depressive episode.)

Susan: "I've just been kind of hanging out at home. I haven't felt like doing much."

Therapist: "You've mentioned that you were feeling drained, and that you have experienced some decreased interest. Have there been other changes that you've noticed?"

Susan: "No, not that I can think of."

Therapist: "What have you noticed about your mood over the past week?"

Susan: "Well, I was feeling pretty upset since last weekend. Jeff was supposed to call me Saturday night but he didn't. That kind of set me off."

Therapist: "I see. How was your mood affected?"

Susan: "I was pretty angry and panicky about it for awhile. I don't think it's bothering me nearly as much now. I'm still in a bit of a funk, though."

Therapist: "I'm getting the sense that you were more bothered by it initially and that things are getting better. Is that accurate?"

Susan: "I think so. But I just haven't felt like doing anything for a few days."

Therapist: "Have you noticed any changes in your appetite?"

Susan: "No, not really. If anything, my appetite has been too good." (Laughs)

Therapist: "How has your energy been?"

Susan: "My energy has always been kind of low."

Therapist: "Would you say there's been a change in your energy recently?"

Susan: "I don't think so."

Therapist: "Have there been any changes in your sleep recently?"

Susan: "No, my sleep has been fine."

Therapist: "Can you say more about how you reacted to the issue with Jeff on Thursday night?"

Susan: "Well, I pretty much freaked out. I thought maybe he wasn't interested in me anymore or maybe that he was planning to dump me. I was crying and pretty upset."

Therapist: "Have things become so upsetting that you've had any thoughts that life isn't worth living?"

Susan: "Oh no, that's not an issue at all."

Therapist: "What about hurting yourself or having thoughts about hurting yourself?"

Susan: "No, no, nothing like that. I'm actually feeling quite a bit better today. Jeff ended up calling me two days ago and it's all sorted out. It was a bit of a misunderstanding, actually. I'm just kind of laying low right now, though. I've been kind of avoiding him. I've done this before. I'm not even really sure why. I was wondering if maybe you might know."

Therapist: "Maybe we can try and understand what's behind that together. Why don't you tell me more about the situation with Jeff and your decision to avoid him right now?"

The example above illustrates the idea that issues that could threaten therapy (such as an evolving episode of clinical depression) typically require immediate attention by the therapist. This will often require the therapist to temporarily shift to a more directive approach, in order to develop a clear understanding of the problem and its potential impact on therapy. This means that the usual patient-driven discourse of therapy may be suspended until the relevant issue is adequately understood. In the example, the therapist asked a number of specific questions about potential depressive symptomatology. When it became apparent that Susan was likely not experiencing an evolving depressive episode (suggested by the lack of change with regard to the neurophysiological symptoms of depression), the therapist clarified any potential safety issues before transitioning back to facilitating observation of Susan's internal world.

In addressing decompensation, it is particularly important to try to ascertain the status of any significant safety issues (e.g., self-harm, suicidal or homicidal thoughts, intent or planning) or urgent medical concerns. Therapy itself may need to be suspended until these issues are adequately understood and addressed. This may involve the patient attending the hospital emergency room (e.g., regarding active suicidal intent or planning, overwhelming self-harm urges, or an urgent medical problem) or the office of her primary care physician (e.g., for a potential nonurgent medical problem) and/or a psychiatrist (e.g., for assessment and treatment recommendations regarding new onset of a psychiatric illness such as major depression, psychosis, or acute anxiety disorder). It may be appropriate to suspend therapy while these issues are being sorted out (e.g., during an acute psychotic episode). If the patient has been admitted to the hospital (e.g., for a major depressive episode), the therapist might choose to visit her during her admission to discuss what happened and to review issues regarding the status of therapy after discharge. Once the problem has been adequately addressed, it is important to meet with the patient with the goal of further clarifying the impact of the situation on therapy. Ultimately, patient and therapist will need to come to a decision about whether restarting therapy would be feasible and appropriate. Restarting therapy may require a renegotiation of some aspects of the treatment contract (e.g., the need for adherence to antipsychotic treatment following a brief psychotic episode). If the patient is unwilling to come to an agreement regarding issues deemed necessary to protect therapy, then the therapist may need to suggest termination, which would ideally involve a number of sessions to work through termination issues. Alternatively, the patient may be unable to continue therapy due to medical illness or due to severe psychiatric illness such as an active psychotic disorder. Again, in cases such as these, suspension of therapy (until the patient is well enough to participate effectively) or termination may be the most appropriate options.

If the decompensation is both due to and limited to an issue intrinsic to the process of therapy itself, it is again important to try to understand the root of the problem. Many of the clinical examples discussed in this text so far involve issues (such as repeated lateness, boundary problems, frustration related to neediness and growing feelings of attachment), which, if left unaddressed, could escalate and potentially threaten the effectiveness of therapy or lead to decompensation. We have discussed how to understand and address a number of these issues according to the four levels of meaning.

One of the more common therapy-related issues that can lead to decompensation is overwhelming anxiety that can result from growing feelings of attachment to the therapist. This often relates to the relationship between growing attachment, neediness, and distress that we have discussed in previous chapters. If left unaddressed, the ensuing distress can lead to the use or escalation of **defense mechanisms**, such as **acting out**,[1] which can threaten therapy. Some common examples of **acting out** are missed appointments, lying to the therapist, self-harm behavior, grossly disordered eating, use of recreational drugs, and dangerous/reckless behavior such as sexual promiscuity. These all reflect unhealthy efforts by the patient to discharge uncomfortable emotions outside of therapy. This can be viewed as circumventing and thereby threatening the therapeutic process.

The therapist may need to repeatedly clarify, confront, and interpret **acting out** in order to ensure the integrity of the patient's therapy. Patients with more severe pathology may continue **acting out** despite these repeated interventions. In such cases, it is important for the therapist to set limits to clarify the expectations regarding these therapy-interfering behaviors, as well as the consequences if the behaviors continue. As setting limits typically

---

[1] **Acting out** is a **defense mechanism** in which intolerable emotions are discharged into unhealthy and often impulsive actions.

involves presenting the patient with a form of ultimatum that threatens abandonment (by withdrawing therapy from the patient if the **acting out** behavior does not desist), this should usually be reserved as a final attempt to preserve the therapy, after other interventions have failed. The following statement is an example of limit-setting for a patient who continues to present to appointments intoxicated despite repeated efforts to address this:

> Unfortunately, I will be unable to help you if you continue to attend your appointments while intoxicated. We've discussed this issue a number of times, yet you've arrived here again today in an intoxicated state. At this point, the only option I have left to try to protect the work we are doing here is to tell you that if you attend again while intoxicated, we will have to end therapy. If that happens, I would be willing to meet with you once or twice more to wrap up and to discuss options that you could pursue to address your marijuana use. Of course, if you ensure that you come here sober from now on, I would be willing to continue seeing you. [2]

Sometimes it will become apparent that a patient who initially seemed to be a favorable candidate for a course of **object relations**–based **psychodynamic psychotherapy** no longer appears to possess the favorable characteristics for this modality (discussed in Chapter Four: Patient Selection) once therapy is

_____

[2] Please note: a patient with substance use problems this severe would likely also require limit-setting around using intoxicants between sessions as well, as this would serve to discharge emotions that should be addressed within therapy.

underway. A poor fit between patient and psychotherapy modality can lead to decompensation. This issue highlights the importance of appropriate initial assessment and biopsychosocial formulation, involving careful attention to the presence or absence of favorable therapy characteristics. In these "poor fit" situations, it is usually prudent to reconsider the diagnosis and your formulation of the primary problem requiring treatment. If there is indeed a poor fit, it is often preferable to consider a change to a more appropriate treatment modality (e.g., to a supportive, psychodynamically informed style of psychotherapy, to a cognitive style of therapy, or perhaps to pharmacotherapy alone). This may involve a transfer to another health professional who is qualified in the particular modality of choice. Again, in such situations, one would ideally meet with the patient several times to discuss the situation and explore termination issues before transfer of care occurs.

In many cases, the patient may struggle somewhat, but may still be an appropriate candidate for **object relations** therapy. A common cause of such struggles is inappropriate pacing of therapy. In this situation, it may be useful to make some adjustments to how you provide therapy, while retaining the overall therapeutic modality. **Object relations** therapy typically involves a shift from discussing issues outside the room to discussing what is going on within the therapeutic relationship in the here and now, typically involving discussion of **transference** issues. If this shift does not occur at a pace that is appropriate and tolerable for the patient (and each patient will have a different capacity with regard to this progression), then overwhelming anxiety and decompensation can result. If you will recall, in Chapter Ten (The Four Levels of Meaning) I suggested the following rule of thumb for the pacing of therapy: trying a few times each session to help the patient experience and interact on one level deeper than the one she is currently comfortable with. Of course, this guideline can be adjusted as needed to minimize the chance of deterioration. As you gain experience with this style of therapy, I suspect your attunement to your patients' anxiety levels will improve. This can help guide your decisions with regard to these pacing issues.

As I had mentioned earlier in the text, it has been my experience that progress in therapy tends to occur in fits and starts. It is not unusual for a patient to experience a few particularly intense sessions characterized by rapid progress, followed by one or more sessions in which progress seems to slow. Perhaps this has to do with the patient's need to slow down in order to process the intensely emotional material addressed in certain sessions. Of course, you should discuss such situations with your supervisor, but I would suggest not becoming too distressed if you notice this type of pattern develop.

CHAPTER FIFTEEN

Structure and How to Use It Therapeutically

What is "structure" in psychotherapy? I use this term to convey the degree of guidance and direction that the therapist provides during the psychotherapy session. As a general rule, increasing "structure" in the session will tend to ease the patient's anxiety. Perhaps you will recall that in Chapter Seven (Beginning the First Session) I mentioned that with very impaired patients I will sometimes begin the session by asking the patient to describe her week, as a way of easing anxiety. This would be an example of providing more structure, compared to beginning the session with silence. As a general rule, the more a therapist talks during a session, the more structure is being provided. When the therapist talks more in the session, this temporarily takes the onus off the patient, which can lead to a reduction in the patient's anxiety. In the previous chapter (Chapter Fourteen: Addressing Possible Decompensation) we saw that the therapist in the dialogue shifted to a much more directive role and asked specific questions to assess for a possible depressive episode. This reflected a shift to providing more structure in the session. A therapist who asks predominantly closed-ended (e.g., "yes or no" or multiple-choice) questions would be providing more structure than a therapist who asks more abstract, open-ended questions.

I would suspect that you may have already employed the therapeutic use of structure intuitively at times in the past. Can you think of any times when you might have done so? What do you think might have led you to do so at the time? I suspect the answer has to do with **projective identification**. A clinician who senses a patient's anxiety will often reflexively infuse structure into the interaction. He or she may become more talkative. Alternatively, the clinician may begin to focus on intellectual/concrete rather than affect-laden matters. In some situations these unconscious decisions by the clinician may happen to be good ones. In others, they might be countertherapeutic. We have discussed a reasoned approach to decision making in such scenarios. Remember, according to the H.O.R.S.E. approach, it is important to consider not only what the patient says and her body language but also your emotional reaction to the exchange before formulating your understanding according to the four levels of meaning (i.e., C.O.S.T.) and determining a corresponding therapeutic response. The benefits of making a concerted effort to go through this process include giving yourself the opportunity to do the following:

1. Understand situations consciously and more thoroughly
2. Decrease the risk of patient mistreatment that can occur by unconsciously identifying with and acting on projected feelings
3. Consciously consider and select from various treatment options

If you notice yourself unconsciously infusing structure into the session, ask yourself: What led me to do that? Once again, initially you may find it easier to do this in retrospect, after the session is over. Then you can consider whether that particular option was the best one for the patient at the time, or whether another option may have been preferable. The use of structure in therapy may be quite appropriate and helpful for patients. The key is to be aware of what you are doing and why you are doing it.

In general, patients with more severe interpersonal pathology often require more structure, at least initially. For example, rather than waiting for the patient to begin speaking, you may decide to begin the session by asking the patient to tell you all about her week. You may decide to use shorter sessions (e.g., 30-minute instead of 50-minute sessions). You may choose to spend more time discussing what is going on outside of the room versus what is going on within the therapeutic relationship (e.g., **transference** issues). You may even choose to work through a workbook (e.g., dialectical behavioral therapy, cognitive behavioral therapy, or other workbooks) together during the sessions. All of these interventions would involve infusing more structure into the appointments. It should be noted, however, that most of these suggestions would reflect a significant departure from "classical" **object relations** psychotherapy, though they may well be informed by the principles of **object relations**.

CHAPTER SIXTEEN

Verbal Attacks on the Therapist

In Chapter Ten (Projective Identification), we saw an example of how patients may launch verbal attacks on the therapist. If you will recall, Susan became irritated with the therapist's **confrontation** regarding her tardiness. She angrily asked: "What's the big deal? Are you paid by the minute or something?" We also saw an example of how to understand such an attack and respond to it therapeutically. Why do verbal attacks happen in therapy? In general, it is often reflective of pathology in our patients' attempts to create and maintain relationships. There can be a multitude of reasons why patients might be angry with the therapist. I will limit my discussion to patient-related reasons, rather than reasons related to actual therapist error or negligence.

Let's consider an example involving our fictitious patient. Imagine that the following conversation takes place during the first session back after a 2-week break from therapy (due to a vacation by the therapist):

  Susan: "How was your time off? You have a nice tan. It must be nice to just be able to up and go on vacation."

  Therapist: "It *is* good to go on vacation. You seem irritated at me. (**confrontation**) Tell me what's going on for you right now." (**clarification**)

  Susan: "Well, while *you* were having a good time, I've had a rough couple of weeks at work. My boss has really been getting under my skin. He just throws all these jobs and deadlines at me, but he doesn't tell me exactly what he wants or how to do all of this stuff."

  Therapist: "You seem angry as you talk about it." (**confrontation**)

  Susan: "Yeah it *is* pretty irritating."

  Therapist: "I imagine it was all the more irritating that this was happening during a break from our sessions. (**confrontation**) What was it like for you that I took time off during this difficult period?" (**clarification**)

  Susan: "It just kind of shows me that I can't depend on anyone to be there when the chips are down. *I'm* supposed to be here every week, but it's okay for *you* to go on vacation for 2 weeks when I need help the most. I don't know why I expected that you would care about my problems anyway."

  Therapist: "You seem quite angry at me for going on vacation, and I'm sorry that you had a difficult time while I was away. This seems to be really affecting the way you're viewing me right now, and I think it's important for us to try to understand that better. Would you be willing to explore that with me at this point?"

Susan: " . . . Well . . . I guess so."

Therapist: "A few weeks back you had mentioned that seeing me was helping you to focus on your feelings, something that you wanted to experience in other relationships as well. Today your view of me seems to have shifted pretty dramatically. You seem to be viewing me as not caring about your problems at all, almost as if you believe that I had *intended* for you to struggle while I was away on vacation. (**confrontation**) Help me understand this because it seems like a pretty radical change." (**clarification**)

Susan: "Sometimes it feels like everyone is just trying to make my life difficult. I guess I get this way sometimes. It's like, if you're not part of the solution, then you're part of the problem."

Therapist: "I wonder if part of you wants me to be the perfect therapist, and when I don't live up to that unattainable ideal you see me as totally uncaring and worthless. I think it's hard for you to experience me as somewhere in between those two extremes." (**interpretation**)

Susan: "I think I'm like that with everyone when things go wrong and I get stressed out. I do the same thing with Jeff, too. Sometimes I just need some time away to deal with being so upset. Then some time goes by and I can act normal around him again."

If you think about the above dialogue, Susan's irritability is quite evident from the beginning. Although the therapist invites her to talk about her frustration directly, she redirects the conversation toward a discussion of her situation at work. The themes she discusses about work parallel the issues in her relationship with the therapist on the fourth level of meaning. She describes her boss as highly demanding, giving her many tasks to do, but providing no guidance whatsoever, much like a parent who has extremely high expectations, yet is distant and inattentive. It is as if her boss tells her what to do and then disappears, much like the therapist did by going on vacation. Susan is experiencing anger related to viewing both her boss and her therapist as demanding, uncaring, and unavailable (this is the active **object representation**). Susan's experience of needing the therapist during the 2-week break from therapy is evident in her comment: "It's okay for *you* to go on vacation for 2 weeks when I need help the most." We could speculate that she reacted to her intolerance of neediness with significant anger (which may have been either conscious or unconscious) toward the therapist for going on vacation and abandoning her.[1]

Notice that the therapist agrees that "It *is* good to go on vacation," instead of becoming defensive (which would likely have led to an escalation of Susan's hostility). This is an example of what I call "rolling with the attack." If you remember to "roll with the attack," I think it will help you to avoid identifying with angry feelings projected by your patients in the heat of the moment. This can sometimes be difficult to do because of intense interpersonal

---

[1] As therapist absences can be difficult for many patients, it is often helpful to repeatedly remind patients of upcoming vacations in the weeks (or even months!) leading up to the break. It can also be helpful for some patients to discuss strategies for dealing with the absence (e.g., journal writing during what would have been the patient's appointment time).

pressure on the therapist to unconsciously act in accordance with the projected emotions. In applying this technique, I may ask the patient, "What is it like for you that I seem so demanding/critical/uncaring/etc.?" This can help the patient develop awareness of the active **object representation**, and how this connects with her affect—anger in this case. In addition, framing your questions or **confrontation** statements in the following way: "You seem to be *viewing me/experiencing me* as . . ." can help patients to develop awareness that their views of themselves and others are representational in nature. This awareness is an important step toward developing the capacity for **mentalization**.

The therapist in the sample dialogue pointed out Susan's shift to an all-bad **object representation**. In the example, Susan was both willing and able to engage in a discussion of her view of the therapist. Unfortunately, this is not always possible when the patient is experiencing particularly intense emotions such as anger. In such situations, it is often preferable to roll with the attack and help the patient to observe and describe her emotional state. You could *try* to encourage integration of the patient's **object representation** at that point (e.g., "You seem to be viewing me in a very negative light. (**confrontation**) Are you able to see any positive qualities in me right now?") However, it can be difficult for a particularly angry patient to engage in this process while distressed, and it may be preferable to explore the inaccuracy of the all-bad **object representation** later (perhaps even during a future session) when the patient has settled and is more willing and able to collaborate in the process.

Patients who have a rigid tendency toward all-good and all-bad **self** and **object representations** (i.e., **partial object relations**) will typically require repeated **confrontation** and **interpretation** of this (often over a period of months, or sometimes even years) to help them integrate and develop conscious awareness of coexistent "good" and "bad" qualities within themselves and others. It can be particularly challenging for severely disturbed patients to develop the capacity to "take back" the disavowed projected emotions or aspects of themselves from the therapist, even when these projections are being returned (via the therapist's responses/interventions) in a sensitive and therapeutic, rather than retaliatory manner. In order to encourage this capacity to take back the projections, it can often be useful to combine **confrontation** with **empathic validation** in one's responses. For example, "Given that you are viewing me as really demanding and critical right now (**confrontation**), I can understand that you would be as angry as you are at me. I wonder if you can describe the anger you're feeling in detail?" (**clarification**) Once the patient's affect has adequately settled, you might ask: "I wonder if you can think of any other ways of looking at my role in the situation?" or "Do you have any ideas as to how *I* might have been feeling during that conversation?" Such questions can help develop the patient's capacity for **mentalization**.

Returning to the sample dialogue, the therapist's apology ("I'm sorry that you had a difficult time while I was away") in this scenario can be understood superficially as an apology for the current situation. On a deeper level, it can be understood as an apology for real or perceived early parenting failures. One might expect, then, that Susan might respond to a heartfelt apology with significant sadness and tearfulness. This sadness may be more intense than expected, as it is reflective of grieving over intense early experiences (i.e., a **transference** reaction). If Susan had reacted to the therapist's apology with significant sadness, then the therapist might have chosen to explore her sad feelings, rather than overlook them in order to focus on her verbal attacks and all-bad **object representation**.

Susan's angry comments in the dialogue superficially reflect her irritation at the therapist for going on vacation. But where did all this anger come from in the first place? And why does the anger seem so out of proportion with the current situation? Again, this likely represents **transference** of anger regarding intensely emotional early childhood experiences. This helps explain why the anger can seem so extreme at times. It is because the intensity of the anger does not relate as much to the present situation as to situations in the past which were likely much more intense for the patient. In the first months and years of life, even small failures in parenting can be perceived by a baby or child as a threat to survival (remember the **paranoid-schizoid position**). In situations of abuse or neglect, the threat may unfortunately be very real. It is therefore not hard to understand that the resulting emotional reactions might be quite overwhelming. This should not be too surprising. We know, for example, that some infants and children even begin to dissociate as a defense against neglectful or abusive caretaking. I would suggest that in situations in which your patients' reactions are more extreme than expected or appropriate, you should consider whether this reflects a **transference** reaction.

If the therapist seems overwhelmed by the intensity of the emotions conveyed (anger in this case), the patient may sense this and choose to "protect" the therapist by diverting to safer topics. She may even drop out of therapy altogether. Thus, the beginning therapist is in a difficult position: his or her lack of experience and consequent discomfort in dealing with intense emotions in therapy can actually lead to patient dropouts and further difficulties gaining experience. This is why it is important to have a simple, easy-to-remember approach for dealing with verbal aggression that you can always fall back on while you are gaining experience: roll with the attack, and go after the affect!

CHAPTER SEVENTEEN

Sadness in Therapy

In the previous chapter I mentioned the sadness patients may experience in therapy that can reflect grieving over early parenting failures. I have observed that this type of sadness often engenders feelings of sadness within me as well via **projective identification**. As a result of this **countertransference** reaction, I often think of this as "true sadness." By contrast, patients can also experience a very different quality of sadness that I think of as "persecutory sadness." This type of sadness is perhaps more accurately described as dysphoria resulting from feeling persecuted by others, by life, or by the world in general. Although this type of affect state can *appear* quite similar to true sadness (e.g., they both may involve tearfulness), persecutory sadness does not tend to engender the same **countertransference** reaction. Rather than feeling sad and moved toward tears myself, I will more commonly become aware of frustration projected from the patient. This type of dysphoria can be thought of as related to the **paranoid-schizoid position** discussed earlier. By contrast, true sadness can be thought of as reflective of the developmentally more mature **depressive position**.

The term **depressive position** was coined by Melanie Klein (1935) to describe the stage in which a child develops the capacity to see others more realistically (i.e., as a person possessing a blend of good and bad qualities) rather than as fluctuating between all-good and all-bad extremes. The depressive sadness that ensues is due to the loss of the idealized yet exciting and jubilant image of an omnipotent caregiver, in favor of the more "depressing" yet realistic notion of a necessarily flawed caregiver. According to Klein's observations, healthy children typically move from a pre-dominantly paranoid-schizoid state to the more mature **depressive position** within the first year of life. Unfortunately, problems may occur that can interfere with this maturational step. These problems may involve serious parenting/environmental issues and/or inherited vulnerabilities. As a result, we see many adult patients who spend much of their time in the **paranoid-schizoid position**. They have not fully progressed to the more mature **depressive position**, which would allow them to relate to and view themselves and others in a more realistic way.

We have already discussed some ways to help our patients spend less time in the **paranoid-schizoid position**. Part of the therapeutic process should involve helping our patients to shift to the more mature **depressive position**. In order to do so, we must help patients to grieve parenting failures and other early losses, and to develop an integrated and realistic view of themselves, their parents, and others in general. This can occur in a symbolic manner by exploring failures within the therapeutic relationship, as we saw in the sample dialogue in Chapter Ten (Projective Identification). Alternatively, patients will often openly discuss and comment on issues related to their upbringing. This type of discussion may lead the patient to an appreciation of how significant early childhood events or repeated early parenting failures (such as abuse and/or neglect) may have contributed to her current emotional and relational difficulties. It can often feel reassuring for patients to hear that "these experiences were not your fault."

When patients experience the healthy sadness characteristic of the **depressive position** (which is often an indicator of progress in therapy), I have typically found it preferable to avoid intervening. Thus, this is one of the few instances in which actively "going after the affect" often seems to detract from the therapeutic process. I would instead suggest allowing the patient some space to experience the emotion without distraction. An exception to this might be if the patient were experiencing this type of sadness near the end of the session. Here I might ask the patient to describe the feeling in detail, so as to help her feel more "together" and to reduce the intensity of the emotion as the appointment approaches its conclusion.

CHAPTER EIGHTEEN

Erotic Transference and Countertransference

As patients' feelings of attachment for the therapist grow, there are often indications that these feelings involve powerful tender/caring as well as sexual feelings. Together, these form what is known as **erotic transference**. When the sexual component of this is exaggerated in therapy, this may reflect the patient's tendency to experience and interpret strong attachment feelings in a predominantly physical way. Perhaps this is not surprising when one considers that very early in life, expressions of love *are* typically very physical (e.g., a mother feeding and holding her baby). This **transference** reaction may come to light through obvious indicators from the patient's speech or behavior. Some patients may begin behaving in an overtly seductive manner. Alternatively, the physical/sexual aspects of **erotic transference** may come to light in a more subtle way. An observant therapist (who is always monitoring for **projective identification** in the therapeutic relationship) may begin to suspect this type of **erotic transference** through attunement to his or her emotional reactions to the patient, rather than from clearly identifiable indications from the patient's speech or behavior. As this suspicion may arise seemingly without obvious or intentional indicators from the patient, it can sometimes be difficult to feel certain enough about it to explicitly address the issue. This can be especially challenging to sort out when the patient is one whom the therapist finds attractive. Add to the picture the possibility that the patient may be consciously unaware of these erotic feelings, and you can see that addressing such issues can become quite complicated indeed.

As you might imagine, experiencing erotic sexual feelings in therapy can be quite uncomfortable for many patients (and for many therapists as well). It can be particularly disconcerting for patients who identify exclusively with a particular sexual orientation (e.g., exclusively heterosexual) to have erotic feelings about the therapist that run contrary to their usual orientation (e.g., experiencing erotic feelings for a same-sex therapist). Many patients find it difficult to separate the tender/caring component from the physical/sexual component of their loving feelings. This could understandably make it difficult to form and maintain mature, platonic, loving relationships. The therapeutic relationship provides a safe context to work through these complicated issues. The following is an example of a possible dialogue related to this topic:

> Susan: "It feels good to be able to talk about my feelings openly."
> Therapist: (Silent, notices a feeling of sexual tension along with prolonged eye contact from the patient.)

Susan: "We talk about some pretty personal things, and I feel like I want be closer to you. I wonder what it would feel like if you were to give me a hug."

Therapist: "You're experiencing some pretty strong feelings about me. (**confrontation**) And that's a pretty normal thing that we can talk about. It's not unusual to want to express those feelings in a more physical way. But that can't happen in this relationship. We can talk about whatever thoughts or feelings you may be having about me, but acting on those feelings in any way, like with a hug, would undermine the work we are doing here, and I wouldn't let that happen."

The above dialogue is one way for a new therapist to handle boundary issues with regard to **erotic transference** of a physical/sexual nature. It reinforces the therapist's role in maintaining boundaries. This can be reassuring for many patients who may experience significant anxiety about their own difficulties with creating and maintaining appropriate relationship boundaries. One of the disadvantages of this approach is that some patients may shut down as a result of preemptive highlighting of the therapeutic boundaries. This may interfere with further exploration of the patient's thoughts, feelings, and fantasies. In other words, emphasizing the boundaries at this point may unwittingly widen the emotional distance in the therapeutic relationship. For this reason, a more experienced therapist might instead invite the patient to talk more about her thoughts and feelings (i.e., about the hug), rather than make a clear statement about the boundaries of the therapeutic relationship at that particular point. Therapist characteristics are not the *only* issue to consider here, however.

The approach described in the dialogue might be preferable for some patients *regardless* of therapist experience and comfort level. Avoiding discussion of sexual fantasies involving the therapist would be prudent for patients who struggle with boundaries and inconsistent reality testing. Again, consideration of the particular patient and situation should reveal which approach, or variant thereof, would be most appropriate and effective.

Throughout this text I have emphasized the importance of careful monitoring of one's emotional reaction to help uncover how **projective identification** may be at work in therapeutic interactions. Careful consideration of the **projective identification** involved in **erotic transference** is particularly important as this is one area in which a therapist's lapse in judgment may have irreversible consequences. The powerful interpersonal pressure to unconsciously identify with the projected material can contribute to therapists becoming convinced that they are falling in love with their patients and/or that they are irresistibly sexually attracted to them. Alternatively, therapists may experience romantic and/or sexual feelings solely as a result of their own needs or issues (i.e., **negative countertransference**). If a therapist were to act on his or her feelings in either of these scenarios, potentially irreparable damage to the patient could result, not to mention the potential damage to one's career. Such situations can be very difficult for new therapists to sort out on their own. It is therefore critically important to discuss **erotic transference** and/or **countertransference** issues in one's psychotherapy supervision.

CHAPTER NINETEEN

Advice in Therapy

The concept of advice-giving in therapy is an interesting and seemingly controversial one. Many of the students I have worked with have been quick to affirm their opinion that it is *never* acceptable to give advice to patients. I am not certain where this notion comes from. Perhaps it stems from concern about giving the wrong advice and about subsequent reprisal. Perhaps it stems from the notion that giving advice may be disempowering or may foster unhealthy dependence on the therapeutic relationship. Alternatively, people may fear that advice-giving represents a slippery slope toward abuse of the power imbalance between therapist and patient. I think that these are all valid considerations when deciding whether giving advice would be prudent in a particular situation. But before discarding advice-giving from our therapeutic toolkit, we must also weigh the potential benefits of giving advice, as well as the possible risks of withholding it.

I think that it is useful to consider the well-trodden analogy of "therapy as reparenting" when thinking about advice-giving. What might good parents do if their child comes to them for advice? Without more information, the best answer is probably "it depends." Do good parents ever give advice? Of course they do! Good parents will often give advice when it is asked for. A parent who refuses to give advice may be viewed as withholding, depriving, or indifferent.

Good parents often give advice even when it is *not* requested of them. Why might they do this? They might do this because they care about their child's well-being and they want to express an opinion about what is best for their child in a given situation. So advice—whether solicited or not—can be an expression of caring. Are there situations in which good parents might withhold advice, allowing the child to make her own decision? Of course there are. Good parents may well decide not to give advice to their child. They might withhold advice when they believe the child would benefit *more* from making her own decision, provided that the child is capable of doing so.

I would suggest to you that the factors involved in deciding when advice is appropriate are very similar in the therapist–patient relationship. Providing advice when it is requested, or even occasionally offering unsolicited advice, can communicate that the therapist cares about the patient. Failure to do so may be perceived as withholding, or as an indication of indifference. Furthermore, on a larger scale, is it not true that the patient is seeing us for "advice" about her emotional health and relationship issues?

Now, before we go too far with this, I am not suggesting that psychodynamic therapists should offer advice about anything and everything. In fact, in my practice, I find that I do not tend to gratify my psychotherapy patients' requests for advice very often. I am, however, offering a counter-argument against what appears to me to be a surprisingly widespread conviction that therapists should *never* offer advice. Advice-giving would certainly reflect a shift to a more supportive stance on the therapist's part. As with any of the techniques that I have described in this text, appropriate use should be determined by a thorough understanding of the particular patient and the particular situation. Such decisions can seem more clear-cut when one considers extreme situations. The decision is often more difficult in situations that lie "in the middle." For example, I suspect that many therapists would have little trouble deciding to give advice if their patient said: "I just received an e-mail saying that I won $1 million. The e-mail said that I have to wire them $2000 by tomorrow to cover the administrative costs of transferring me the money. I'm thinking I'll do it today when I get home. What do you think?" Conversely, I suspect most therapists would be comfortable withholding advice if their patient (a professional stock market trader) asked: "So, what do you think, should I sell Global Oil short? Or should I buy a few hundred thousand shares of Midwest Textiles?" It is the situations that lie in the middle that can be more challenging to sort out. Should I offer my patient advice about what to say or do in certain difficult interpersonal situations? Should I offer my patient advice about continuing versus discontinuing a problematic friendship? Should I offer my patient advice about how to manage a stressful work situation? What about quitting a job? What about getting a divorce? The decision about whether to provide advice in these situations can be much more difficult.

When faced with such situations, I will often consider the issues described in the good parenting analogy discussed above. The following is a list of questions that may be relevant to your deliberation:

- Is the patient *asking* me for advice?
- What does this request mean with regard to the four levels of meaning?
- If the patient is not asking for advice, is this a situation in which I would prefer to offer unsolicited advice as an expression of caring and because I have a strong opinion about what would be best for the patient?
- Is this patient *capable* of arriving at a good decision on her own?
- What would the likely emotional impact on the patient be if I were to withhold advice in this situation?
- Would there be value in stepping back and allowing the patient to learn and grow from making and then redressing a small mistake?
- Is the patient about to make a poor choice that may lead to significant problematic (albeit avoidable and foreseeable) consequences?
- Do I have good advice to offer?[1]
- Does this decision need to be made urgently or can it await further deliberation and discussion?

I think that these are all potentially important questions to consider when deciding whether giving advice is appropriate.

---

[1] Note: It is often *very* difficult to be certain of this, even when the answer may *seem* evident. One of the reasons for this is that we are often relying solely on our patient's possibly distorted or inaccurate view of a situation.

My advice to you is to look at each situation carefully and make a reasoned decision either way, rather than rigidly dismissing advice-giving altogether as a matter of principle.

Let's look at a couple of examples illustrating how to apply some of these ideas in hypothetical situations involving our fictitious patient Susan. In this first example Susan is soliciting advice regarding a "middle-of-the-road" issue: the decision about whether to end her romantic relationship with her partner Jeff.

> Susan: "So I'm thinking of ending it with Jeff. He never listens to me and I'm feeling pretty fed up with it . . . What do *you* think I should do ?"
>
> Therapist: "Well, my first reaction is that is this all seems quite sudden. You haven't mentioned thoughts about ending your relationship with Jeff before. (**confrontation**) Help me understand what led up to this." (**clarification**)
>
> Susan: "Like I said, he doesn't listen to me. He's too pre-occupied with his own life. That's not the kind of relationship I want. I want a relationship with someone who actually cares what's going on for me and takes the time to listen."
>
> Therapist: "It sounds as if you're experiencing Jeff as distant and disinterested. And you're suggesting that your needs aren't being met." (**confrontation**)
>
> Susan: "Are you saying that I should leave him then?"
>
> Therapist: (Noticing a sense of urgency and interpersonal pressure from Susan.) "I haven't given you any advice either way. As we've been talking about this, I've noticed a sense of urgency from you to have me give you advice

about a situation that I have very little information about. I wonder if you have any thoughts about what that might be like for me?" (**clarification**)

Susan: "Hmm . . . I guess I wasn't really thinking about that. I guess it is kind of an unfair question."

Therapist: "The idea of possibly ending your relationship is understandably pretty stressful. I think at times of stress it can be harder for you to put yourself in someone else's shoes and consider the impact of what you say and do." (**interpretation**)

Susan: "I think that's true. I know I can sometimes be insensitive when I'm panicked. Then I feel bad about it later . . . but I'm still stuck with this decision."

Therapist: "I guess I can understand that you would want me to give you advice about what to do. Having someone else decide might relieve some of the pressure you're feeling to try to figure this out on your own." (**interpretation**)

Susan: "It has been pretty intense. I've been mulling it over since last night."

Therapist: "Well, I'd certainly be willing to talk it through with you. We can sort through it together, though I think that ultimately *you* are in the best position to make this decision. Not only that, but I also feel confident that you're capable of deciding for yourself. Why don't you take me through it in detail?" (**clarification**)

This dialogue is an example of a middle-of-the-road situation in which the patient is requesting advice and the therapist refuses to provide it. Let's think about this exchange according to the four levels of meaning. Susan is requesting advice from the therapist about her dilemma regarding whether to continue her relationship with her boyfriend Jeff. This would be the concrete or superficial level of understanding. What does the dialogue tell us about how Susan is viewing Jeff? The therapist confronts Susan with a statement regarding her active **object representation** pertaining to Jeff: viewing him as distant and disinterested (it is difficult to know whether this view is realistic). In terms of how Susan is viewing herself (i.e., her **self representation**), she seems to be seeing herself as rejected and devalued by her partner, but she is aware that she has the power to end the relationship if she so chooses (i.e., she is not viewing herself as completely helpless). The affects connecting the **self** and **object representations** appear to be irritation, ambivalence, and a sense of urgency (all of which are corroborated by Susan's urgency and insistence that the therapist provide advice). The therapist seems to recognize that these aspects of Susan's emotional state are being projected. Rather than identifying with and unconsciously acting on these affect states (e.g., by becoming irritated and perhaps offering an impulsive or glib answer to her question), the therapist asks Susan to reflect on the situation and on the feelings her behavior may be leading the therapist to feel. This requires that Susan consider her own emotional state and also imagine the emotional state of the therapist. This intervention can help to engage and develop Susan's capacity for **mentalization**.

How can we understand this dialogue in terms of the fourth level of meaning—what Susan is communicating about her relationship with the therapist? There seem to be a couple of possibilities here. Which possibility is more likely would depend in part on Susan's recent experience of the therapeutic relationship.

It would seem possible that Susan has noticed significant differences between her relationship with her boyfriend Jeff and her relationship with the therapist. She is noting aspects characteristic of the therapeutic relationship which she perceives to be missing in her romantic relationship—that is, "someone who actually cares what's going on for me and takes the time to listen." This may be leading Susan to question her relationship with Jeff. Alternatively, Susan may be displacing her current feelings about the therapist—whom she may perceive as "distant and disinterested"—onto her boyfriend Jeff, leading her to question the romantic relationship. As is sometimes the case, further **clarification** would be needed to help the therapist identify which (if either) of these possible hypotheses is accurate. Then a decision could be made about how to best address the relevant issue.

By declining Susan's request for advice in this situation, the therapist is demonstrating that one need not respond to projected urgency from others in interpersonal interactions. The therapist is modeling the capacity to defer a decision until later, despite significant external pressure. He or she does not reject Susan's request out of hand, but rather suggests a collaborative effort to work through the issues together. It is also clear that Susan will ultimately be responsible for making the decision, and the therapist reassures her regarding her ability to do so. All of this models a mature, considered response to pathological **projective identification** (involving Susan's projected urgency, ambivalence, and aggression).

Now let's consider an example in which the therapist offers unsolicited advice. Let's pick up part of the way through another session. Susan is talking about impulsively relocating to a city in another state (a decision that would bring her therapy to a premature end) secondary to frustration with her employer regarding an issue at work:

> Susan: "I'm just so fed up with him. I go out of my way to do everything he wants and he just expects more and more. It never ends. I don't know how I ended up doing his personal errands. I'm an office manager, not his personal slave! I'll show *him* though. I'm quitting and moving to Chicago. The firm has an office there and they've posted a position identical to mine. I'm sure I'll get it. I've got lots of work experience. I'm sick of this city anyway."

> Therapist: "You seem quite annoyed with the situation. (**confrontation**) Why don't you take me through it in detail?" (**clarification**)

> Susan: "What's to go through? The solution is pretty simple. And if things are meant to be with Jeff, then it'll still work out as a long-distance relationship."

> Therapist: "Well, moving away might well end the conflict with your employer. And it might leave him scrambling to find someone to fill your position at the firm. What do you think would be the impact of moving impulsively like that on *your* life?" (**clarification**)

> Susan: "It would mean moving all my stuff, which would mean renting a moving truck. I'd have to find a new place, and a new job. I guess it would be pretty hard on my relationship with Jeff . . . and I'd have to stop coming here. I don't know! Why is life so difficult!?"

> Therapist: "I think this idea of moving, as tempting as it may seem, is a geographic solution to an emotional and inter-personal problem. (**interpretation**) I think making an

impulsive decision at this point would create a major upheaval in your life, in the ways that you have identified. You also mentioned that it would bring a quick end to the work that we're doing here, and I think that would be very unfortunate. What do you think about holding off on this decision until we can work through it in detail together?"

Susan: " . . . I know that logically you're probably right. I just want him to feel what *I'm* feeling."

Therapist: "That's an interesting observation. Why don't you tell me more about that?" (**clarification**)

In the dialogue above, the therapist is offering unsolicited advice about Susan's temptation to make an impulsive move in response to interpersonal/work issues with her employer. Susan appears to be in the throes of the **paranoid-schizoid position**. She is in a panic and sees only one solution to her problem. The therapist suggests deferring a decision until her emotional intensity dissipates and she is able to consider all aspects of the situation. The therapist's advice reflects concern about the possible consequences of an impulsive move to a different city. One of these consequences would be a premature end to Susan's therapy. Thus, the advice also serves to protect Susan's treatment. This dialogue also illustrates that it can be both acceptable and appropriate to shift to a more supportive approach (as advice-giving is considered a supportive technique) when the patient is in crisis or when the patient's therapy may be in jeopardy.

CHAPTER TWENTY

Self-Disclosure

Like advice-giving, self-disclosure is an issue with which beginning therapists may struggle. It can be tempting to adopt a black-and-white view with regard to such issues (this would constitute a form of **splitting**, by the way) in order to ease anxiety about sorting through potentially complicated decisions. As in the last chapter, I would suggest that you avoid rigidly dismissing self-disclosure as a therapeutic option without first considering the patient and situation. The issue of self-disclosure typically arises as a result of patient inquiry, though the therapist may also choose to disclose personal information if it is deemed beneficial for the patient's therapy.

We indirectly touched on the issue of patient requests for self-disclosure in Chapter Thirteen (Neediness in Therapy). Susan had commented on the clear imbalance in the relative amounts of disclosure within the therapeutic relationship. This example illustrates how the patient's neediness often intensifies as feelings of attachment grow within the therapeutic relationship. This commonly leads to efforts by the patient to establish a more equal balance of power. This may lead to requests that the therapist disclose personal information. With patients who are able to tolerate discussions on the fourth level of meaning, I will usually encourage an exploration of the process described above. But what of the request for disclosure itself? Should you answer the question? Should you sidestep it? In deciding whether to answer a personal question, the following are some key issues that I will typically consider:

1. How does this patient manage boundaries?
2. What kind of information is being requested?
3. How do I understand the request in terms of the four levels of meaning?

Initially, I was going to list the first question last. But then I realized the importance that I typically place on this issue, and I decided it should go first. In general, I would be reluctant to disclose personal information to patients who have poor personal and relationship boundaries. With such patients, maintenance of boundaries within the therapeutic relationship is of paramount importance, for the reasons reviewed in Chapter Six: The Value of Rules and Boundaries. One of the important ways that patients learn how to create and maintain their own boundaries (both interpersonal boundaries and boundaries with regard to the patient's sense of self) is by abutting boundaries created and maintained by the therapist. If boundaries are a significant problem for a particular patient, I would typically require compelling answers to questions two and three in order to warrant disclosure.

The following brief dialogue illustrates an example of refusing to disclose personal information:

> Susan: "I'm not sure what's okay and what's not okay to ask you—like more personal questions about you."
>
> Therapist: "You can ask me anything you like. I may choose not to answer certain questions, though."
>
> Susan: "Sometimes I wonder where you live, what your house looks like, what colors you chose in your house . . ."
>
> Therapist: (Silent)
>
> Susan: "Do you have any children?"
>
> Therapist: "I think it's natural for you to be interested in knowing more about me. I don't actually discuss the details of my home life with any of my patients, though. Tell me about what's behind your curiosity about that." (**clarification**)
>
> Susan: "I don't know . . . I just think you would make a good father."
>
> Therapist: "That's kind of you to say. Tell me more about that." (**clarification**)
>
> Susan: "Oh, I don't know . . . you seem kind of easy-going. You listen . . . and you don't seem to get mad or upset. You're always the same . . . consistent, I guess."

In the example above, Susan requested permission to ask more personal questions of the therapist. This will not always occur. Sometimes patients will ask very personal questions without any warning. Alternatively, patients may ask gradually more and more personal questions in an escalating fashion, to find out where the boundaries are and whether boundaries even exist.

In the example above, Susan did not get angry about the therapist's boundaries. Rather, we could speculate that the therapist's adherence to boundaries in this instance reinforced her perception of the therapist as "consistent." This demonstration of boundary stability may have been perceived as quite reassuring. Patients will often either consciously or unconsciously pick up on such demonstrations of boundary-setting. It would not be unusual for a patient such as Susan to return the next week and talk about an instance in which she was able to make or maintain clear boundaries in a relationship herself—without necessarily making a conscious connection with what had transpired in therapy the previous week. This is an example of one way that progress in therapy can occur, as the patient unconsciously internalizes aspects of the therapist.

When is it appropriate to disclose information about oneself in therapy? For patients who have demonstrated an ability to create and maintain appropriate boundaries, selected personal disclosures can provide a type of "normalizing" reassurance (e.g., "I must be okay if my therapist reacted like I did in a similar situation") and can lead to a deepening of therapeutic rapport through **identification** with the therapist. This shared experience can represent a common historical link, allowing the patient to recognize valued qualities of the therapist within herself. However, just as avoiding self-disclosure reflected an adherence to boundaries in therapy, it should be noted that revealing personal information conversely reflects a loosening of therapeutic boundaries. For that reason, I tend to be very selective regarding my use of this technique.

The decision about disclosure also depends on the type of information that is being requested. In general, I would be more apt to disclose my thoughts or feelings about the patient, as opposed to specific details about my personal life. The therapist's thoughts or feelings about the patient are often relevant to the therapeutic process. I would not typically view disclosure of such material as a boundary transgression, but rather as a useful facet of the therapeutic relationship that can help move therapy forward. We saw an example of a request for disclosure of this type in Chapter Thirteen (Neediness in Therapy) when Susan asked what the therapist was writing about her. Let's look at a similar example, as this issue tends to come up quite frequently:

Susan : "You must think I'm pretty much nuts."

Therapist: (Remains silent. Waits to see where this is going.)

Susan: "I mean, I'm kind of all over the place, aren't I? One minute I'm breaking up with my boyfriend, the next I'm picking up and moving to another city because I'm pissed off at my boss. But you never really criticize me . . . I'm curious what you think my problems are?"

Therapist: (Noticing Susan's appreciative tone, conveying her feelings of attachment.) "It sounds as if you feel that I've been helpful to you. You seem to be feeling appreciative of that." (**confrontation**)

Susan: "Yeah, I guess I am. But I notice you didn't answer my question."

Therapist: "That's true. I suppose I'm in a bit of mystery as to the connection between your appreciative feelings and your question about my intellectual understanding of your issues. I wonder if at the root of your question is a desire to know how I *feel* about you. But I imagine you might feel more comfortable asking me about my

130

thoughts rather than my feelings about you." (**interpretation**)

Susan: (Appears mildly anxious.)

Therapist: "I also believe you already know the answer to *that* question. I think you know that I care about you, as I care about all of my patients."

Susan: (Silent for several seconds. Appears on the verge of tears.) ". . . I didn't like that last part so much."

Therapist: "Which part is that?" (**clarification**)

Susan: "The part about *all* of your patients. I don't really like to think about you seeing other patients. I guess in a way I like to think of myself as your only patient, or maybe that I'm somehow special, you know, different from your other patients."

Therapist: "I can understand that. I suspect that has to do with some of the imbalances in this relationship. Like the fact that I see many patients, whereas you see only one therapist. It's understandable that this imbalance is uncomfortable for you, given that you are experiencing positive feelings about me. Can you say more about those feelings?" (**clarification**)

In this dialogue the therapist comments on Susan's caring and appreciative feelings. Susan responds by inquiring about the therapist's intellectual formulation of her difficulties, rather than by direct inquiry about the therapist's feelings about her. The therapist interprets her use of **intellectualization** as a defense against anxiety related to her feelings of attachment. The therapist then comments on experiencing caring feelings for Susan while noting the limits of those feelings. Susan's response ("I didn't like that last part too much") suggests that she feels disappointed in reaction to these limits. This leads the therapist to empathize with Susan's discomfort regarding the imbalances in the therapeutic relationship. The therapist could then ask Susan to further describe her feelings about the imbalances. This would reflect **identification** with Susan's projected discomfort about discussing her caring feelings. Instead, the therapist helps Susan to see that the discomfort she is experiencing is tied to her positive feelings about the therapist. This is followed by an invitation for Susan to describe these positive feelings in more detail.

Requests for disclosure about the therapist's personal life can be difficult to sort out in the heat of the moment. This is because there is often a projected pressure to respond immediately. As illustrated in the first dialogue in Chapter Eighteen (Advice in Therapy), it may be useful and therapeutic to defer a decision until you have had time to think about the issues clearly. (For example, "I'm actually not sure whether to answer your question at this point. Your question raises some important issues to do with the boundaries in this relationship. I think perhaps we need to explore those issues first.") This can allow you more time to consider the situation using the H.O.R.S.E. and C.O.S.T. approaches.

Coming up with examples of appropriate disclosure (solicited or not) about the therapist's personal life was a difficult task for me in writing this chapter. I think this is because I disclose so infrequently about my personal life, since boundary issues tend to be such an integral part of treatment for many patients. One situation in which I may disclose, however, has to do with therapist absences (e.g., due to vacations or conferences). As a general rule, I try to give all of my patients as much advance notice as possible when I will be away. With patients for whom boundaries are not a key issue (i.e., those who have consistently demonstrated good boundaries within the therapeutic relationship), I may disclose my vacation or conference destination if this information is requested. With other patients, I might not gratify requests for further details. Of course, patients will notice the therapist withholding such details. This will typically lead to a discussion of the imbalances within the therapeutic relationship and the patient's reaction to this. Thus, more rigid maintenance of boundaries with such patients actually promotes *further* exploration of boundaries as a treatment issue.

CHAPTER TWENTY-ONE

Gifts in Therapy

In this chapter, we will discuss how to understand and address a situation in which the patient wishes to give the therapist a gift. This can be an awkward situation for many new therapists. Accepting a gift requires a loosening of therapeutic boundaries. Declining a gift can feel as if the therapist is trouncing upon the patient's appreciative, caring feelings. In order to avoid this dilemma, some therapists adopt a black-and-white policy regarding gifts in therapy. Some therapists might choose to almost always accept gifts. Others may decide to essentially never accept gifts. If you have read the previous chapters, I think you can probably guess what I am going to suggest as an alternative to such predetermined and rigid policies: considering each particular patient, gift, and situation according to the four levels of meaning in order to determine a preferred course of action.

As accepting a gift involves therapeutic boundaries, I would suggest a similar approach to the one that we discussed with regard to requests for self-disclosure. Specifically, I would suggest asking yourself the following three questions:

1. How does this patient manage boundaries?
2. How appropriate is the gift as a small token of appreciation for therapy?
3. How do I understand the gesture in terms of the four levels of meaning?

As in the case of self-disclosure, there are a number of issues to consider. All other things being equal, I would be less likely to accept a gift from a patient for whom boundaries are a significant problem. In addition, by their very nature, some gifts are clearly inappropriate as a small token of appreciation (e.g., giving the therapist a house) regardless of the patient's economic resources or consideration of cultural norms. For patients who are less economically fortunate, even seemingly small gifts might represent an overwhelming economic stretch and may therefore be inappropriate on that basis.

In some situations it may be quite evident that the preferred course of action is to politely decline the gift (e.g., "Although I certainly accept and value the feelings of appreciation that lie behind this gift, I'm afraid I can't actually accept the gift itself because of how important the boundaries are in this relationship") and then discuss the significance of the gift and the impact of the therapist's refusal in detail with the patient. In other situations, it will seem quite clear that the appropriate course of action is to graciously accept the gift (e.g., "Thank you very much. This is really very kind and thoughtful of you") and again discuss the situation in detail with the patient.[1] Many situations however, will lie in the middle, and the preferred course of action may initially seem unclear. Furthermore, **projective identification** is often involved in gift-giving. As a result, the therapist will often experience a great deal of pressure to accept the gift without a second thought. In such situations, it is useful to remember that this is not an either/or situation. A third option almost always exists: deferring the decision until later. Let's break down one of these in-the-middle situations further using a sample dialogue with our fictitious patient Susan:

> (Susan stands up from her chair just as her appointment has come to an end. She reaches into her purse and produces a small wrapped gift that is approximately the size of a ring box. She reaches out to hand the gift to the therapist.)
>
> Susan: "Oh yeah, before I go I wanted to give you this as a way of saying thank you for all your help. I really appreciate everything you've done for me and this is just a little something that I picked up. It's no big deal. I just thought you might like it."
>
> Therapist: (Does not take the gift from Susan.) "Oh my ... that's very thoughtful of you, Susan. I'm afraid that you've taken me a bit by surprise, presenting me with this after our session has ended. I wonder if . . . ."

---

[1] Conspicuously displaying the gift (e.g., on the therapist's desk) during the current and subsequent sessions can be a useful tactic for gently prodding the patient to discuss the gift's significance and meaning.

Susan: (Interrupting) "It's no big deal if you don't want it, I can always take it back."

Therapist: "I was just going to say that we unfortunately can't give this issue the time and attention that it deserves and needs today. I was wondering if you wouldn't mind bringing the gift in with you next time so we can talk about it at the beginning of the next session?"

Susan: "I don't have to bring it if you don't want it."

Therapist: "As I had mentioned, this is a very thoughtful gesture, but you *have* caught me a bit off guard with the timing. Presenting one's therapist with a gift is a bit of an unusual situation that requires more time than we have today. So at this point, I'm not able to say whether I will be accepting the gift. What I *can* say, however, is that I'm very grateful and accepting of the feelings of appreciation behind the gift and I would like you to bring the gift in with you next time so we can discuss the significance of it. Would that be okay?"

Susan: "Sure. I hope I didn't do something wrong. I feel kind of awkward."

Therapist: "This *is* a bit of an awkward situation, mostly because we don't have more time today to discuss things further. But situations like this are an important part of the work that we're doing here together. And we have as much time as we need ahead of us to talk about it, starting at our next session."

Susan: "Okay, see you then."

This dialogue illustrates that a therapist need not respond to the **projective identification** to reflexively accept a gift. In this situation, the gift was presented after the session was over, leaving very little time to process the situation and determine an appropriate course of action. Furthermore, the gift was wrapped, and therefore the appropriateness of the gift itself was still in question. As a result, the therapist decided to validate the patient's feelings of appreciation but did not accept the gift at that point in time. If the gift had been unwrapped, the therapist might have accepted the gift, declined the gift, or suggested bringing the gift to the next appointment (e.g., if the therapist was still uncertain about accepting or declining the gift). This decision would depend on the therapist's mental deliberation regarding the three questions we had discussed earlier. Given the strong emotions commonly invested in gifts within therapy, it is particularly important in such situations to remain courteous and respectful, despite possibly experiencing a **countertransference** reaction (perhaps involving discomfort and irritation) to the manner and timing of the gift presentation. Let's continue with this example and see what happens at the next session:

Susan: (Presents the therapist with the gift—a paperweight.) "You've got a lot of papers on your desk and I thought this might help keep some of them from flying around."

Therapist: "It certainly will. Thank you. That's very kind and thoughtful of you. Tell me all about how this gift came to be." (**clarification**)

Susan: "Well, I feel like you've helped me a lot. You're always listening to me and helping me sort through my feelings about people and my personal life. I felt like I wanted to do something nice for *you* for a change."

Therapist: "You're talking about some of the imbalances in this relationship that we've discussed before. But something is different today. You don't seem to be viewing those imbalances in a negative light." (**confrontation**)

Susan: "No, I guess not . . . you know, after the last appointment I wasn't even sure if you were going to accept it."

Therapist: "Tell me about that." (**clarification**)

Susan: "I felt kind of uncomfortable at the end of the session last week. I thought about it during the week, and I think I kind of sprung it on you at the last second because I was feeling uncomfortable about giving you the gift earlier during the session. I guess I was pretty worried about how you would react to it, and whether or not you would accept it."

Therapist: "How were you hoping I would react?" (**clarification**)

Susan: "Well, first of all, I was hoping you would accept it. It would be pretty embarrassing if you didn't. And then I guess I was hoping that you would like it."

Therapist: "I do like it, Susan. The gift represents your positive feelings for me. So I can understand that it would be important to you that I accept it. Otherwise it might feel as if I was rejecting your caring feelings. (**interpretation**) I think you're probably right about how you understood your decision to present me with the gift right at the end of the last session. That way, no matter what happened, you could make a quick exit."

Susan: "Exactly." (Smiles)

Therapist: "If indeed the gift represents your caring feelings for me, it would seem that having the paperweight here at my office is a way for you to leave me with a reminder of your positive feelings, even when you're not here. (**interpretation**) Perhaps you can tell me more about that?" (**clarification**)

In this dialogue, the therapist accepted the paperweight from Susan and proceeded to explore the significance of the gift with her. They discussed the motivation for the gift, Susan's reaction to the last appointment, her uncertainty about the therapist possibly declining the gift, the gift as a symbol of Susan's positive feelings for the therapist, and her intention that the gift serve as a **transitional object**[2] for the therapist. In situations in which the therapist declines the gift, the themes mentioned above are all still relevant and important to discuss. It would be particularly important, however, to sensitively explore Susan's reaction to the therapist's refusal in some depth, as the refusal of a gift can be particularly upsetting for many patients. Because of the intense emotions that may be involved, many patients will initially minimize the impact of the refusal (e.g., "It's no big deal. Don't give it a second thought"). Rather than attempting to interpret this at the time of the refusal, it can sometimes be preferable to revisit the issue at a later session, when emotions may be less intense. At a subsequent session, the patient may be more able to appreciate and discuss how the refusal affected her. She may also be more prepared to accept and make use of an **interpretation** of her defensive need to minimize the initial impact of the refusal.

---

[2] In childhood, this is the blanket, toy, or other inanimate object that a child imbues with the caregiver's soothing qualities. Other mementos can serve a similar function involving attachment figures in adulthood.

CHAPTER TWENTY-TWO

Putting It All Together:
A Sample Session

In this chapter, let's look at a longer dialogue to try to simulate the flow of an actual psychotherapy session. Hopefully this will give you an idea of what an actual psychotherapy session may look like. I have also included some thoughts and observations from the therapist's perspective to shed some light on the therapist's thought processes. As you read through it, try to think about what is going on according to the four levels of meaning. In particular, try to piece together an understanding of the interaction according to the fourth level (what is being communicated with regard to the relationship with the therapist). Can you identify Susan's **self** and **object representations** and the affect linking them? Hopefully this will help to consolidate some of the material that we have already covered. You may find that it also introduces a few new ideas and techniques that you might find useful in your own practice.

(Susan arrives on time for her appointment. The therapist greets her in the waiting room and they enter the office to begin the session. Over the past several months Susan had been discussing her frustrations about both her employer and her boyfriend Jeff. These frustrations were paralleled by Susan's experience of the therapist as withholding and rejecting. As a result, therapy had been focusing on confronting and interpreting Susan's tendency to experience herself and others as either "all good" or "all bad" (as discussed in Chapter Sixteen: Verbal Attacks on the Therapist). Recently Susan appears to be developing insight into her tendency to experience inaccurate and polarized views of herself and others. She has been demonstrating evidence of a new capacity to see herself and attachment figures as possessing both good and bad qualities simultaneously. In the past few weeks Susan has focused less on experiencing the therapist as rejecting/withholding, and more on her feelings of appreciation for therapy. The session begins with the therapist waiting silently...)

Susan: "I felt really good after the last session. I thought it was pretty positive. I think I've just been feeling more relaxed overall lately."

Therapist: (Decides to remain silent and observe where Susan chooses to take the session, rather than, for example, asking about Susan's affect at this point.)

Susan: "... I bumped into an old high school friend earlier this week. Well, we were sort of friends. I mean, we weren't close or anything. Anyway, I had some free time and we decided to go for coffee. So I was kind of expecting to feel nervous and scared of being rejected, like I usually do in these kinds of situations. But I didn't. I felt pretty calm, even when the conversation sort of slowed down a couple times when no one was talking."

Therapist: "So just as you're feeling more comfortable with silence here, you were more relaxed in *that* situation as well." (Interpreting the parallel between Susan's increasing comfort with silence in therapy and her similar experience with her acquaintance earlier in the week.)

Susan: "Yeah. I was thinking about it later and I realized that during those awkward moments when no one's talking I've always either felt really panicky and self-critical, thinking that I've got nothing to offer, or else I'd get kind of irritated and I would be convinced that the person was thinking something critical about me—but they weren't letting me in on it. But I didn't do that this time. I just sat there and kind of observed the situation without judging myself or Julie, my friend. I remember thinking while it was happening that it was kind of like when I'm sitting here and neither of us is talking."

Therapist: (Remains silent, seeing no need to interrupt this introspective moment. Quietly notes the parallel between the current moment of silence and Susan's last sentence. The therapist notes feeling relaxed during the pause, and suspects that this indicates that Susan is likely also feeling comfortable, despite the period of silence.)

Susan: "You know, that whole episode made me think about how often I've thought people were rejecting me or attacking me when that wasn't really the case. Like all the times I've given you a hard time. I remember that time when you went on vacation. I kind of felt like you were intentionally abandoning me and that you should have known better. That was pretty unfair of me. And I shouldn't have taken it out on you like that. You should be allowed to have a vacation just like anybody else. I kind of took it like a personal rejection. But I know it wasn't . . . I've been pretty nasty to you at times. I feel pretty bad about that. I think that's partly why I wanted to give you a gift. To show you that I appreciate you putting up with that kind of stuff from me."

Therapist: (Aware of caring feelings from Susan in response to her comments. Wonders if Susan's comments reflect integration of good and bad within her **object representations**, or whether alternatively she may have switched to an idealized perception of the therapist. Observes that Susan's comments seem consistent with a potential shift toward the **depressive position**.) "It sounds as if you're feeling regret for the way you behaved those times when you experienced me as rejecting you." (**confrontation**)

Susan: "I guess I am. Those weren't my best moments. I still can get pretty angry sometimes, like with Jeff. And it can be hard to slow down and observe myself when I get really angry at him. But I think I'm getting better at it. When I get upset, it's always been so tempting to see him as nothing but a jerk. But I'm trying not to do that. I try to remember that he's the same guy who's super nice and funny and considerate most of the time. The same with my boss. Sometimes it's so tempting to think he's just the biggest loser. But I'm trying to check myself when I feel that temptation, and I try to remember what you and

I keep talking about, you know, about seeing people as "all good" or "all bad" when I get really upset. The reality is my boss *can* be pretty annoying and inconsiderate at times. But at other times, he can be pretty understanding. He doesn't have to be so cool with me leaving early on Thursdays to come here, for example. So I just try and remember stuff like that when I get irritated at him, and it helps me to avoid freaking out."

Therapist: "You've described what sounds like a number of positive changes that you've noticed in the past while. (**confrontation**) I wonder if you thought about telling me about these things over the past week?" (**clarification**)

Susan: "I thought about it a couple of times over the past week but mostly this morning. I wanted to talk about it."

Therapist: "What is it like telling me?" (**clarification**)

Susan: "I guess it feels okay. I'm not uncomfortable about it or anything."

Therapist: "How were you hoping I would feel hearing about these successes that you've experienced?" (**clarification**)

Susan: "I hadn't really thought about that . . . I guess I want you to feel good about it too because you've helped me with all this stuff."

Therapist: "I do feel good about it, Susan. It sounds as if you'd like me to feel proud of you, and I do." (Notices an intensification of Susan's affect involving a heightening of caring feelings as well as feelings of sadness.)

Susan: "I don't think my parents ever said that they were proud of me growing up." (Appears on the verge of tears.)

145

Therapist: (Silent . . .)

Susan: " . . . I always worked really hard in school. But it seemed like it was just never good enough. Maybe I was always looking for them to be proud, but I think I've accepted that that's not going to happen. Maybe it's too late for that now. I don't know. Maybe I would've become a different person if I'd had that. But I don't think I need that from them anymore."

Therapist: "That sounds sad, Susan."

Susan: "Yeah . . . You know, I don't think I've ever really felt sad about it growing up. I felt angry a lot at my parents, though. Especially my mom. Sometimes it seemed like no matter what I did, she'd find a flaw. But at other times she would go to the ends of the earth to do something nice for me. She was kind of all over the map that way. There wasn't a lot of middle ground with her. She was all about extremes. She's still kind of like that sometimes, but I think it's settled a bit over the years. And then there's my dad. He was always kind of in his own world. He just wasn't around as much as I would have liked. I think he cares in his own way but he's just kind of distant about it . . . No wonder I'm messed up, huh!?" (Attempts a laugh.)

Therapist: "It seems that as you're developing a better understanding of your issues, you are also thinking about how you became the person that you've become. You're describing some things that weren't ideal for you growing up. It sounds as if you felt like your needs weren't met as well as they might have been. And it *is* sad to think about that. That feels like a loss for you." (**confrontation**)

Susan: "Yeah, I guess it does. It's weird, you know I actually felt happier at the beginning of the session."

Therapist: "Tell me what you're feeling right now, Susan." (**clarification**)

Susan: "I'm feeling kind of sad. I think it's a bit odd that I'm more comfortable with my therapist than I ever have been with either of my parents. But the truth is, I think that you know me better than either of them do. I mean the real me—on the inside. They may know more of the details of my life and stuff, but that's not what I'm talking about . . . It's kind of weird to say this but if I'm having a rough week, I don't call my parents or think about them too often. I think of coming here and telling you about it. It's kind of stabilizing for me. I still get frustrated with you sometimes, but overall I feel like this is my space where I can talk about anything."

Therapist: (Silently notes the evidence of improved **object constancy** suggested by Susan's comments.) "You *do* feel a lot of freedom here." (**confrontation**)

Susan: "It's nice to be able to talk about whatever is on my mind and feel like that's okay. I'd like all my relationships to be more like that."

Therapist: "That *would* be nice . . . (Glances at the clock.) . . . I see that we are out of time for today, Susan."

Susan: "Okay. See you next week then."

Therapist: "Yes. See you then."

CHAPTER TWENTY-THREE

What Is Progress in Therapy?

In Chapter Three (The Big Picture) we discussed some of the common areas of progress in **object relations** therapy. In subsequent chapters we have gone over some suggestions for inciting change in a number of these areas through the therapeutic relationship. This has generally involved using the H.O.R.S.E. and C.O.S.T. approaches as a framework for understanding the problems introduced into the therapeutic relationship by the patient. We have discussed a number of common ways that these problems can present in the day-to-day practice of psychotherapy, as well as some examples and discussion of how to address them.

We have reviewed some ways to help patients develop their capacity for self-soothing and spend less time in the **paranoid-schizoid position**. We have also discussed how to manage neediness in therapy and how to help patients tolerate their neediness and growing feelings of attachment. We have emphasized the importance of boundaries within the therapeutic relationship and discussed how this can help patients develop a clearer sense of personal and interpersonal boundaries. We have also discussed the importance of processing the losses involved in problematic parenting and how to help patients develop a more realistic, integrated view of themselves, their parents, and others. We have reviewed how to help patients focus on their caring feelings rather than focusing solely on negativity. We have also covered how to understand and manage **erotic transference** and **countertransference** that can arise in the therapeutic relationship.

In the previous chapter, a number of Susan's comments suggested that she had made progress in several of the areas described in the paragraph above. She described a decreased tendency toward the **paranoid-schizoid position**. She also described an increased capacity for observing her affect, even during times of stress. She was able to describe her feelings in the moment, including positive, caring feelings for the therapist. She also described experiencing feelings of regret regarding her mistreatment of the therapist in the past. This is suggestive of a shift to the **depressive position**. It is also suggestive of an improved capacity for **mentalization**. As she described her relationship with attachment figures (including the therapist and her parents) she described coexistent positive and less favorable qualities, suggestive of integration of her previously polarized **object representations**. This capacity was not evident at the beginning of therapy, as Susan experienced attachment figures using predominately **partial object relations**. Lastly, Susan described being able to retain a mental and emotional connection with the therapist's frustrating and satisfying qualities, even between sessions. This is suggestive of improvements with regard to her capacity for **object constancy**. If these areas of progress are sustained over time, this would suggest that Susan has accomplished the treatment goals identified at the outset of her therapy. Remember, the primary treatment goal was to help her shift from use of partial to predominantly **whole object relations**. Secondary treatment goals were improved capacity for self-reflection/**mentalization** and improved control of intense affects. These all contribute to the overarching goal of improving Susan's relationships with herself and with others.

Once the patient has developed the capacity to have a mature, healthy, caring relationship with the therapist, it often becomes apparent that she is no longer attending therapy because she "needs to." The sense of urgency, intense distress, and over-whelming need-that reflected the **paranoid-schizoid position** ear-lier in therapy-may now be a rare, or very brief occurrence. The earlier attempts at pathological **projective identification** may no longer occur or may be less frequent and intense. Instead, ongoing attendance seems to reflect healthy enjoyment and satisfaction derived from the therapeutic relationship. Patients who began therapy using predominantly **partial object relations** may now demonstrate a sustained capacity for relating to themselves, the therapist, and others using **whole object relations**. Those patients who already had the capacity for **whole object relations** at the outset of therapy may experience less intrapsychic conflict, less anxiety, and may tend to avail themselves of healthier, more mature **defense mechanisms**. Evidence of change should also be evident in the patient's life outside of the therapeutic relationship. For example, the patient may begin to select and maintain heal-thier relationships outside of therapy. Once there is evidence that the patient has accomplished the treatment goals, and that these are sustained, rather than transient changes, then the time has come to begin working toward termination.

I think that the outcomes described above reflect an ideal that we should all strive for. In my experience, however, the changes that occur in actual practice tend to vary from patient to patient. Although very favorable outcomes can and do occur, I think it is somewhat unusual to see a miraculous sweeping transformation involving all of the changes described in the last paragraph. Some patients may make good progress in one area, but little progress in others. Other patients progress in a number of different areas, but the magnitude of each change may be small. Unfortunately, this is a field in which poor, even tragic outcomes can occur. Humility and embracing one's role as a lifelong learner are crucial to the practice of psychotherapy. Just as we would like our patients to recognize and accept their limitations, so too should we accept our own limitations as therapists. Psychotherapy supervision is the ideal context for the necessary ongoing critical appraisal of one's effectiveness as a therapist.

CHAPTER TWENTY-FOUR

Termination and Other Therapy Endings

Working through issues related to termination is an important step in the therapeutic process. It can be very helpful for the patient to gradually work through letting go of the therapeutic relationship and to address the impact of this. A patient's ability to move beyond the therapeutic relationship can be seen as a symbolic reflection of her ability to fully separate from her parents and successfully begin to lead an autonomous and mature life.

Clearly, not all endings to therapy involve the termination process described above. Patients may suddenly stop attending therapy and may not respond to the therapist's attempts to inquire about and address this. This can be seen as quitting therapy, rather than as termination per se. When a patient misses a therapy appointment, I will typically consider a few options. First, I may call the patient during her designated appointment time. If she is not available to discuss the absence, I may leave a message noting the absence and asking the patient to please call and confirm her next appointment. Alternatively, I may wait for a few days before calling to see if the patient calls. Finally, I may not call at all. Instead, I may wait to see if she attends her next scheduled appointment. The option I will pursue will depend on the particular patient and how I understand her absence in light of the four levels of meaning, along with consideration of any relevant safety issues in more severely disturbed patients. If the patient has missed a few sessions in a row and has not responded to my attempts to reach her by telephone, I may choose to write her a letter inquiring about her absence and clarifying the steps that would be required to reinitiate therapy. In this letter, I will often include a statement similar to the following: "If I do not hear from you within the next three weeks, in other words by September 14, I will assume that you do not wish to continue therapy with me and will instead continue to follow up with your general practitioner, Dr. Jones." I may send a copy of this letter to the general practitioner involved in the patient's care, to try to ensure continuity of care, in case the disruption in therapy reflects a significant problem or decompensation. If the patient responds to my attempts to reach her, I will meet with her to try to understand and address whatever led to the disruption. We will discuss whether continuing therapy would be appropriate and beneficial from both of our perspectives. This discussion may involve a renegotiation of the terms of the treatment contract.

A patient may suggest termination of therapy for any number of reasons. The reason may be unrelated to the therapeutic process (e.g., a geographic move). Alternatively, the patient's reason may be reflective of issues going on within the therapeutic relationship. The patient may feel that she has accomplished her personal

therapeutic goals. Alternatively, she may feel completely dissatisfied with therapy, or anything in between. As you might expect, my
general approach here would be to try to understand the stated
reason(s) according to the four levels of meaning. As a result of this
analysis, I may agree with the patient's reasons for termination, or
I may disagree and express my opinion that the patient needs and
would benefit from continued therapy. Can you see that suggesting that she continue with therapy can convey that I care
about the patient and that I feel hopeful that she can benefit
from treatment? It should be made clear, of course, that the
ultimate decision lies with the patient and that your opinion
stems from your concern for the patient's well-being and therapeutic progress.

The therapist may suggest discontinuing therapy for reasons
similar to those mentioned in the previous paragraph. The reason
may be unrelated to the therapeutic process (such as changing jobs),
or it may stem from an issue within the therapeutic relationship. In
Chapter Fourteen (Addressing Possible Decompensation) we discussed some situations in which significant deterioration in the
patient's functioning may necessitate termination of therapy. We
also discussed how **acting out** in therapy can sometimes lead to
termination. **Negative countertransference** is common in such
situations, and it may unconsciously sway the therapist's decision
to terminate. It is important to work through the reasons for
termination with the patient, hopefully with adequate time to help
her deal with the fact that ending therapy was not her idea. Working
through these issues may sometimes lead to the decision to refer the
patient to another therapist or to other appropriate resources.

I would suggest spending some time in the weeks or months
leading up to termination discussing what it will be like for the

patient to be ending therapy, as well as reviewing what occurred during the course of treatment. This may involve a review of the areas of progress that we discussed in previous chapters, and any other significant issues that the patient has worked through (e.g., grieving the loss of a loved one). In addition, this review may involve a discussion of any of the patient's criticisms of the therapy process. Part of this discussion may involve an acknowledgement of the therapist's limitations. This relates to the **depressive position**, which, as we discussed in Chapter Seventeen (Sadness in Therapy) involves the loss of the idealized image of the caregiver in favor of a more realistic, integrated view. In addition, I have found that patients often respond particularly well to a review of their strengths prior to ending therapy. This can help mitigate feelings of uncertainty related to the stress of losing the therapeutic relationship. This may also help reduce the possibility of regression to a prior pathological pattern. Having adequate time to process the significant loss of the relationship is one of the most important reasons why termination should be discussed and worked through so far in advance.

Regardless of whether a specific termination date is preplanned, the final appointment may involve discomfort for the patient, the therapist, or both. Let's take a look at this using the following dialogue from the last few minutes of Susan's final therapy appointment:

> Susan: "I can't believe there's only a few minutes left and this is our last appointment. It's kind of surreal."
>
> Therapist: "It *is* hard to believe that it's been almost 2 years since you began therapy."
>
> Susan: "It sure is. I'm going to miss coming here. I feel like you've helped me a lot. I'm in a totally different place

than when I first started seeing you. But it's still going to be kind of weird not having this appointment to come and talk about things."

Therapist: "It's been my pleasure having you as a patient, Susan. You've done a lot of hard work over the past 2 years. Over the past several weeks we've talked about a number of positive changes you have created both within yourself and in your life in general. You've made great strides in your ability to view yourself and others in a balanced way during times of stress. You're also much more able to use self-observation as a way of regulating your emotions and being more present in the moment. You've developed a better sense of boundaries in relationships and this has helped you sort out some of the difficulties you were experiencing with Jeff and at work. Those are some pretty impressive accomplishments. I know you are more than capable of managing without me from here on in. At the same time, you will always be able to think back to your memories of therapy. And it sounds like for the most part, they'll be fond ones." (Smiles)

Susan: "Yes, they will be . . . for the most part." (Laughs)

Therapist: "Well, we're going to have to wrap up. I want to wish you all the best." (Shakes hands with Susan.)

Susan: "Okay. Thanks again."

Therapist: "Take care."

In this dialogue the therapist briefly reviews some of the key areas of progress during the course of Susan's therapy. In addition, the therapist provides some reassurance in response to

Susan's expression of uncertainty about the future. Lastly, the therapist makes a comment to reinforce Susan's sense of **object constancy**. You will notice that the therapist shook hands with Susan at the end of the appointment. This reflects maintenance of professional boundaries with a patient who had some difficulties with boundaries during the course of her treatment. You may be wondering whether it is ever appropriate to hug a patient at the end of therapy. As with most of the issues that we have discussed in this text, I would not view a hug at the end of therapy as inherently "right" or "wrong." Again, the decision about the appropriateness of a goodbye hug should really be determined by what the hug would mean with regard to the four levels of meaning for the particular patient. For example, I would be unlikely to hug a patient who continues to experience significant boundary issues. Similarly, a hug may be inappropriate with a patient for whom **erotic transference** has been an unresolved or incompletely resolved issue in therapy. Often the issue of a goodbye hug does not come up unless the patient specifically requests one (e.g., "Is it okay if I give you a hug?"). Some patients will attempt to give their therapist a goodbye hug without fore-warning, however. Such situations can indeed be awkward for both patient and therapist. I would suggest that you decide in advance of the last appointment whether agreeing to a goodbye hug would be appropriate for your particular patient. This may even be an issue that you may wish to discuss in advance with the patient. These steps should help to prevent you from making a misguided, impulsive judgment call as a result of **projective identification** during the final moments of your patient's therapy, when there may be little or no time to discuss the issue further.

CHAPTER TWENTY-FIVE

Object Relations Concepts and Cognitive Therapies

In Chapter Two (The Big Picture) I stated that one of the particular strengths of **object relations** therapy lies in helping patients with integration. I think it is therefore only fitting that we discuss integration of **object relations** concepts with other therapeutic modalities.[1] In previous chapters we discussed an approach to understanding patients and their difficulties according to the basic principles of **object relations** therapy. In this chapter, I would like to elaborate on the utility of these ideas for understanding and addressing patient **resistance** within a cognitive therapy model. I am using the term "cognitive therapy" broadly to encompass time-limited, problem-focused, structured, often

---

[1] For an excellent integrated approach to the main forms of **psychodynamic psychotherapy**, I refer you to Glen Gabbard's *Psychodynamic Psychiatry in Clinical Practice*.

manualized forms of therapy—the prototypical example being cognitive-behavioral therapy (CBT)—that are not specifically based on psychodynamic theory. Cognitive therapies will often involve "homework" that the patient must complete as part of the treatment. As with any treatment, problems may develop that limit the patient's response to therapy. I am hopeful that the **object relations** concepts that we have discussed will provide therapists from other orientations with a useful complementary framework for understanding and addressing these problems, in order to promote the best possible patient outcomes.

In his book *When Panic Attacks*, cognitive therapist David Burns writes that approximately 75% of his anxious patients are "sweeping some problem or feeling under the rug" (p. 315). He goes on to further discuss unconscious issues, describing them as "some problem or feeling you're avoiding because you don't want to upset anyone or hurt their feelings" (p. 316). Dr. Burns provides a number of case examples to help readers identify and address unconscious difficulties in his chapter entitled the "Hidden Emotions Technique" (pp. 313–329).

In their CBT manual *Clinicians Guide to Mind over Mood*, authors Christine Padesky and Dennis Greenberger refer to issues related to the "therapy relationship" as a possible cause for patients' lack of improvement in response to treatment (p. 29). Drs. Padesky and Greenberger remark that a "therapist may have difficulty maintaining empathic rapport with a client who is describing a struggle that closely parallels a current life experience for the therapist" (p. 29). I think you will agree that this sounds very much like the concept of **negative countertransference** that we discussed earlier. The authors go on to describe various patient beliefs that can interfere with compliance in therapy. These include the following: "My therapist will criticize me," "If I show my therapist what I am thinking she will know I'm crazy," "If my therapist really cared, she would know how tough it is for me and not ask me to do more" (p. 35). The examples in this and the previous paragraph suggest that there is indeed common ground between CBT and **psychodynamic psychotherapy** in understanding difficulties that can arise, even if the terminology used to describe these difficulties is different. These examples point to the relevance of unconscious issues, as well as the importance of attending to **transference**, **countertransference**, and **resistance** within the therapeutic relationship, as these can all influence treatment outcome regardless of therapeutic modality. In particular, the quality of the therapeutic relationship has been shown to be an important independent predictor of psychotherapy treatment outcome (Martin et al., 2000).

Earlier in this text, we discussed the H.O.R.S.E. approach to identifying what the patient is communicating. The C.O.S.T. approach then provides the therapist with a framework for understanding these communications according to four possible levels of meaning. I am hopeful that these concepts can be used to complement and enrich treatment within virtually any therapeutic model. In previous chapters we discussed how to understand and address a number of common issues that arise in **psychodynamic psychotherapy**. Some of the issues we discussed were lateness, missed appointments, scheduling problems, and boredom in therapy. I think most would agree that these issues are relevant to the practice of virtually all forms of therapy. As we have already discussed an approach to understanding and addressing these common issues, I will not revisit this here. Rather, I would like to focus on an issue that we have not yet discussed that I think is more pertinent to cognitive therapy.

One important distinction between cognitive therapy and **psychodynamic therapy** is cognitive therapy's emphasis on homework as part of the treatment plan. Drs. Padesky and Greenberger noted in the aforementioned clinician's guide that: "If the client routinely does not complete assignments, noncompliance can be a focus in therapy" (p. 35). I would like to discuss how to understand and address **resistance** with regard to this common problem that can arise in cognitive therapy. Let's look at a sample dialogue involving a fictitious patient (Stanley), who is engaged in individual cognitive behavioral therapy for panic attacks:

(Stanley has attended each of his four appointments thus far in his 16-session course of CBT for panic attacks. He did not complete his assignments prior to the last two appointments.)

Therapist: "Perhaps at this point we should turn to reviewing your thought records from the past week."

Stanley: "Oh, I . . . I actually didn't do them."

Therapist: (Notices a feeling of irritation in response to Stanley's passive noncompliance) "I see. I notice that this is the third week in a row that you have not completed the assignments. I'm concerned that if we don't try to understand what's behind this, it could seriously affect your treatment, and you have told me how much these panic attacks really affect your life. Could you help me understand what you think is making it difficult for you to complete the assignments, Stanley?"

Stanley: "I'm not sure. I plan to do it when I leave here. But then it just doesn't happen. I don't really know why." (Slumps somewhat in his seat.)

Therapist: (Observes a feeling of helplessness in response to Stanley's answer and body language.) "Well, perhaps you can tell me how you feel about doing the thought records. I realize that you haven't done them on your own at home, but we've completed a couple here together. How did you find completing the thought records here with me?"

Stanley: "I don't really know. I guess it was okay. I'm not sure it really helped much though. I'll try and do it for next time."

Superficially, Stanley is attending his appointments and claims that he is making an effort, as indicated by his statement: "I'll try and do it for next time." Nonetheless, it seems that he is merely "going through the motions" of therapy. Stanley's words, actions, and body language all seem to convey a passive, helpless, and defeated **self representation**. The therapist in the dialogue ascertains this by observing Stanley's body language, listening carefully to what Stanley is saying and noting the emotions that Stanley is projecting, namely helplessness and irritability. Although there is no clear evidence of this in the dialogue, we could further speculate that Stanley may be experiencing the therapist as assertive and dominating, which would contrast with his experience of himself. The information about Stanley's **self representation** stems from careful observation of what is occurring within the therapeutic relationship via **projective identification**. This understanding can now help the therapist to weigh options as to how to address the situation in order to promote the desired outcome: effective participation in therapy, ultimately leading Stanley to relief from his troublesome panic attacks. Let's see how the rest of the interaction unfolds:

Therapist: "I wonder if you're feeling like there's no point, as if no matter what we do, things won't get any better?" (**confrontation**)

Stanley: "Yeah, maybe."

Therapist: "I imagine that might leave you feeling pretty frustrated with yourself, with me, and with the whole situation." (**confrontation**)

Stanley: ". . . I think that's true, it *is* pretty frustrating. And on top of it all, my wife is on my case to get my act together . . . like I can just snap my fingers and make these attacks stop! Not to mention my boss—do you think he has any clue what a panic attack even is? I'm sure he just thinks I'm slacking off of work."

Therapist: "It certainly sounds like you feel caught in the middle of everyone's expectations. And I'm a part of that too, expecting you to complete the assignments each week. (**confrontation**) I can understand how that might seem irritating, given everything you're dealing with."

Stanley: "It shouldn't irritate me. I know you're just trying to help me. You're the only person I've told about all that stuff. It actually feels good to get it off my chest."

Therapist: "Well, I am glad you did because not only is it creating an obstacle to feeling better, but I suspect you've felt quite alone with all of this. I think it's also possible that your thoughts and feelings about these issues may have a lot to do with the panic attacks themselves. (**interpretation**) What do you think about going through a thought record about your interactions with your wife or your employer?"

Stanley: "I guess if it is related to my anxiety, why not?"
Therapist: "Which of the two relationships would you like
   to go over first?"

In the dialogue above, the therapist simultaneously confronts
Stanley regarding his frustration about himself, the therapist, and
the world in general. In doing so, the therapist addresses the
second, third, and fourth levels of meaning (others, self, and
therapist). This leads Stanley to reveal his frustrations with
regard to his home and work environments. The therapist then
focuses specifically on the fourth level of meaning, empathically
confronting Stanley's irritation with the therapist. This
confrontation leads Stanley to take back his projected hostility
and begin to experience a more realistic, integrated view of the
therapist as a well-meaning, yet necessarily imperfect caregiver.
Stanley's comments also reflect an improvement in therapeutic
rapport. This improved rapport, along with the new insights
regarding potential issues underlying Stanley's panic attacks (i.e.,
tension with his spouse and employer) led to the therapist's suggestion to further discuss these issues via thought records. Stanley
agrees to this suggestion. Although the outcome in this session
appears to be favorable, it is quite possible that Stanley's passive-
aggressive interaction style may persist, requiring similar interventions in the future to help facilitate continued progress. Although
his interpersonal style is clearly self-defeating, his passive opposition in various spheres of his life may provide Stanley with a subtle,
likely unconscious sense of triumph over the wishes and expectations of others.

Although the topic of integrating psychodynamic and cognitive therapies is a broad one, I hope that the above example

illustrates that these two psychotherapeutic models are not mutually exclusive and in fact can work together synergistically. In the next and final chapter we will look at how **object relations** concepts and principles can be of use in a variety of clinical contexts.

CHAPTER TWENTY-SIX

Object Relations Concepts in General Follow-Up

In the preceding chapters we reviewed some concepts, principles, and practical aspects of **psychodynamic psychotherapy** from a predominantly **object relations** perspective. I am hopeful that this material will be as helpful for you as it has been for me as you develop experience as a therapist. In this concluding chapter, however, we will explore how these same skills and ideas can enrich the care you can provide in virtually any clinical setting. I will be discussing some thoughts related to mental health assessments, inpatient follow-up, and outpatient follow-up.

Mental health assessments demand a broad and multifaceted skill set. Clinicians must not only be very familiar with the features of mental illnesses, they must also be skilled at the arts of inquiry, observation, and inference. There is so much verbal and nonverbal information coming at the interviewer during an assessment that it can sometimes be overwhelming and difficult to know what to focus on. Throughout this text, I have emphasized the importance of attunement to one's emotional reaction to the patient, as this can provide a window into the patient's affect state and relationship patterns. This is a powerful diagnostic and therapeutic skill that you can bring to bear in your assessment interviews. Considering **projective identification** (using the H.O.R.S.E. and C.O.S.T. approaches) in your interviews can reveal a tremendous amount of information about how the patient interacts with others. It also gives you very useful information that can guide empathic comments to help speed and deepen the development of therapeutic rapport. As you see more and more patients, you will develop a "**projective identification** database" of sorts that can provide a very sensitive reference, honing diagnostic acuity and bolstering your skills for understanding the person as a whole, rather than merely as a collection of diagnostic criteria.

The principles and skills that we have discussed can also be very useful in inpatient settings. Such settings are often populated by individuals experiencing disorders such as schizophrenia, bipolar disorder, or recreational drug-induced psychosis. At first blush, it may be difficult to envision how psychotherapy concepts and skills might be useful for individuals who have had such a significant break from reality. Clearly, however, the rapport-building skills discussed in the previous paragraph are perhaps even more important in this challenging population. In addition, your skills for understanding the patient's story with regard to the four levels of meaning can be very useful for treating patients with psychotic disorders. The content of delusions and auditory hallucinations typically speaks volumes about a patient's experience of herself and the world around her.

Let's consider an example of a patient who believes the government is spying on her using surveillance equipment that she believes is implanted within her. How can you understand the deeper meanings of this? The patient is projecting intolerable feelings of malevolence and persecution onto the government. This suggests a desire to protect goodness within herself from the perceived evil outside. This sounds a lot like the **paranoid-schizoid position**, doesn't it? The government's decision to spy on *her* in particular can be seen as a grandiose element of the delusion. This grandiosity can be viewed as defending against powerful underlying feelings of inadequacy and unimportance. The fact that surveillance equipment is purportedly implanted within the individual speaks to the fragile boundaries of self that this patient experiences. When one understands the issues underlying the content of the psychotic symptoms, it becomes very difficult *not* to feel compassion for this person's plight. This understanding of the internal issues that the patient is experiencing can now inform and guide your efforts to develop a collaborative therapeutic alliance that may lead to improved overall treatment adherence. You may also be in a position to help the patient better understand and cope with a very confusing and frightening perception of the world.

I work in a hospital-based adult psychiatric outpatient setting. My clinical work generally involves assessment and short-term and long-term follow-up of individuals experiencing mood, anxiety, and personality disorders. I have observed that many of the same emotional and relationship difficulties that bring patients into therapy are at play regardless of the specific disorder or treatment type. Most of the issues that we have discussed with regard to **object relations** psychotherapy (e.g., missed appointments, intolerance of neediness, boundary issues, **projective identification, transference, resistance, erotic transference,** and **countertransference**) will also arise in other treatments such as interpersonal therapy for depressive illness, cognitive-behavioral therapy for panic disorder, dialectical behavioral therapy for borderline personality traits, lithium treatment for bipolar disorder, supportive therapy for an adjustment disorder, or exposure and response-prevention for obsessive-compulsive disorder. Hopefully, the material that we have covered will enrich your work and provide some guidance for addressing these issues when they arise, helping to foster a collaborative, caring, and truly therapeutic relationship with your patient, because in my humble opinion, that's what it's all about.

References

Abernethy, B. (1988). Dual-task methodology and motor skills research: Some applications and methodological constraints. *J Hum Movement Stud* 14:101–132.

Ahnert, L., Gunnar, M. R., Lamb, M. E., and Barthel, M. (2004). Transition to child care: Associations with infant-mother attachment, infant negative emotion, and cortisol elevations. *Child Dev* 75(3):639–650.

American Psychiatric Association. (2000). *Diagnostic and statistical manual of mental disorders* (4th edition, text revision). Washington, DC: American Psychiatric Association.

Anisman, H., Zaharia, M. D., Meaney, M. J., and Merali, Z. (1998). Do early-life events permanently alter behavioral and hormonal responses to stressors? *Int J Dev Neurosci* 16(3–4):149–164.

Beatson, J., and Taryan, S. (2003). Predisposition to depression: The role of attachment. *Aust NZ J Psychiat* 37(2):219–225.

Blunt Bugental, D., Martorell, G. A., and Barraza, V. (2003). The hormonal costs of subtle forms of infant maltreatment. *Horm Behav* 43(1):237–244.

Burns, D. D. (2006). *When panic attacks: The new, drug-free anxiety therapy that can change your life.* New York: Morgan Road Books.

Chugani, H. T., Behen, M. E., Muzik, O., Juhasz, C., Nagy, F., and Chugani, D. C. (2001). Local brain functional activity following early deprivation: A study of postinstitutionalized Romanian orphans. *NeuroImage* 14(6):1290–1301.

Cloninger, C. R., Svrakic, D. M., and Przybeck, T. R. (1993). A psychobiological model of temperament and character. *Arch Gen Psychiat* 50:975–990.

Etkin, A., Pittenger, C., Polan, H. J., and Kandel, E. R. (2005). Toward a neurobiology of psychotherapy: Basic science and clinical applications. *J Neuropsych Clin N* 17:145–158.

Freud, S. (1905). *Three essays on the theory of sexuality*. Standard edition of the complete psychological works of Sigmund Freud, 7:121–245. London: Hogarth Press, 1953.

Freud, S. (1933). *The dissection of the psychical personality*. Standard edition of the complete psychological works of Sigmund Freud, 22:57–80. London: Hogarth Press, 1964.

Gabbard, G. O. (2004). Long-term psychodynamic psychotherapy: A basic text. Arlington, VA: American Psychiatric Publishing, Inc.

Gabbard, G. O., and Westen, D. (2003). Rethinking therapeutic action. *Int J Psychoanal* 84:823–841.

Graham, Y. P., Christine, H., Goodman, S. H., Miller, A. H., and Nemeroff, C. B. (1999). The effects of neonatal stress on brain development: Implications for psychopathology. *Dev Psychopathol* 11:545–565.

Gunnar, M. R. (1989). Studies of the human infant's adrenocortical response to potentially stressful events. *New Dir Child Dev* (45):3–18.

Guttentag, R. E. (1989). Age differences in dual-task performance: Procedures, assumptions and results. *Dev Rev* 9:146–170.

Hartmann, H. (1952). The mutual influences in the development of ego and id. *Psychoanal Stud Chil* 7:9–30.

Hertsgaard, L., Gunnar, M., Erickson, M. F., and Nachmias, M. (1995). Adrenocortical responses to the strange situation with disorganized/disoriented attachment relationships. *Child Dev* 66(4):1100–1106.

Høgland, P., Bøgwald, K., Amio, S., Marble, A., Ulberg, R., Sjaastad, M. C., Sørbye, O., Heyerdahl, O., and Johansson, P. (2008). Transference interpretations in dynamic psychotherapy: Do they really yield sustained effects? *Am J Psychiatry* 165(6):763–771.

Horvath, A. D., and Symonds, B. D. (1991). Relation between working alliance and outcome in psychotherapy: A meta-analysis. *J Couns Psychol* 38:139–149.

Jung-Beeman, M., Bowden, E. M., Haberman, J., Frymiare, J. L., Arambel-Liu, S., Greenblatt, R., Reber, P. J., and Kounios, J. (2004). Neural activity when people solve verbal problems with insight. *PLoS Biol* 2, E97.

Kernberg, O. S. (1984). *Object relations theory and clinical psychoanalysis.* Northvale, NJ: Jason Aronson (original work published in 1976).

Kernberg, O. S. (1992). *Aggression in personality disorders and perversions.* New Haven, CT: Yale University Press.

Klein, M. (1935). A contribution to the psychogenesis of manic-depressive states. *Int J Psychoanal* 16:145–174.

Klein, M. (1946). Notes on some schizoid mechanisms. *Int J Psychoanal* 27:99–110.

Ladd, C. O., Owens, M. J., and Nemeroff, C. B. (1996). Persistent changes in corticotropin-releasing factor neuronal systems induced by maternal deprivation. *Endocrinology* 137:1212–1218.

Martin, D. J., Garske, J. P., and Davis, M. K. (2000). Relation of the therapeutic alliance with outcome and other variables: A meta-analytic review. *J Consult Clin Psychol* 68(3):438–450.

Padesky, C. A., and Greenberger, D. (1995). *Clinician's guide to mind over mood.* New York: The Guilford Press.

Piper, W. E., Azim, H. F., McCallum, M., and Joyce, A. S. (1990). Patient suitability and outcome in short-term individual psychotherapy. *J Consult Clin Psych* 58:475–481.

Raine, A., Phil, D., Mellingen, K., Liu, J., Venables, P., and Mednick, S. A. (2003). Effects of environmental enrichment at ages 3–5 years on schizotypal personality and antisocial behavior at ages 17 and 23 years. *Am J Psychiatry* 160:1627–1635.

References

Sanchez, M. M., Ladd, C. O., and Plotsky, P. M. (2001). Early adverse experience as a developmental risk factor for later psychopathology. *Dev Psychopathol* 13:419–449.

Schore, A. N. (2001). Effects of a secure attachment relationship on right brain development, affect regulation, and infant mental health. *Inf Mental Hlth J* 22:7–66.

Shefler, G., Dasberg, H., and Ben-Shakar, G. (1995). A randomized controlled outcome and follow-up study of Mann's time-limited psychotherapy. *J Consult Clin Psych* 63:585–593.

Siegel, S. M., Rootes, M. D., and Traub, A. (1977). Symptom change and prognosis in clinical psychotherapy. *Arch Gen Psychiat* 34:321–329.

Sloane, R. B., Staples, F. R., Cristol, A. H., Yorkston, N. J., and Whipple, K. (1975). *Psychotherapy versus behavior therapy.* Cambridge, MA: Harvard University Press.

Squire, L. R. (1987). *Memory and brain.* New York: Oxford University Press.

Viinamaki, H., Kuikka, J., Tiihonen, J., and Lehtonen, J. (1998). Change in monoamine transporter density related to clinical recovery: A case-control study. *Nord J Psychiatry* 52:39–44.

Westen, D. (1999). The scientific status of unconscious processes: Is Freud really dead? *J Am Psychoanal Assoc* 47:1061–1106.

Westen, D., and Gabbard, G. O. (2002a). Developments in cognitive neuroscience, I: Conflict, compromise, and connectionism. *J Am Psychoanal Assoc* 50:53–98.

Westen, D., and Gabbard, G. O. (2002b). Developments in cognitive neuroscience, II: Implications for theories of transference. *J Am Psychoanal Assoc* 50:99–134.

Glossary

(Please note: defense mechanisms are indicated by an asterisk)

*Acting out: an immature defense mechanism in which intolerable emotions are discharged into unhealthy and often impulsive actions.

*Altruism: a mature defense mechanism in which a person puts the needs of others before the needs of the self.

Attachment theory: one of the four main theoretical frameworks of psychodynamic psychotherapy. Attachment theory posits that children are biologically driven to maintain close proximity to their caregiver. The child develops internal working models for future relationships based largely on the qualities of the child–caregiver relationship. Problems therein can lead to suboptimal attachment styles, difficulties with mentalization, and concordant relationship difficulties in adulthood.

Borderline personality organization: pertains to individuals who tend to view themselves and others as either "all good" or "all bad," experience identity disturbance, are impulsive, experience transient impairment in reality testing, have poor capacity for mentalization, and tend to use immature defenses such as splitting and projective identification (Gabbard, 2004, p. 31).

Glossary

Clarification: an invitation from the therapist for the patient to elaborate, in order to promote a better understanding of an issue.

Confrontation: a statement or question by the therapist that directs the patient's attention to something that is being avoided or minimized.

Countertransference: the therapist's total emotional reaction to the patient.

Defense mechanism: a typically unconscious mental process that protects the individual from anxiety-provoking, unacceptable, or otherwise distressing psychic experiences. Often classified as immature, neurotic, or mature defenses.

*Denial: an immature defense mechanism in which an uncomfortable aspect of external reality is disregarded.

Depressive position: a mature developmental stage (compared to the paranoid-schizoid position) characterized by the capacity for whole object relations and an appreciation of one's destructive potential in relationships.

*Displacement: a neurotic defense mechanism in which an individual shifts the focus of intense feelings from the original object or idea to another similar object or idea that is less distressing.

*Dissociation: an immature defense mechanism involving a drastic change in personal identity or mood state to avoid distress (e.g., can occur in dissociative fugue and dissociative identity disorder).

Ego psychology: one of the four main theoretical frameworks of psychodynamic psychotherapy. Focuses on intrapsychic conflict between the ego, id, and superego as a result of competing sexual and aggressive drives. Such conflicts create anxiety, which is quelled through the use of defense mechanisms.

Empathic validation: a statement from the therapist that demonstrates attunement with the patient's emotional experience.

Erotic transference: a type of positive transference involving both tender/caring and sexual loving feelings.

***Humor:** a mature defense mechanism in which something unpleasant is viewed in a comedic light in order to manage the situation in a less distressing way.

***Idealization:** an immature defense mechanism (related to splitting) in which an individual inaccurately views another as "all good" in order to avoid experiencing ambivalence and subsequent distress (e.g., anxiety or contempt).

***Identification:** a neurotic defense mechanism in which an individual takes on qualities of another.

***Intellectualization:** a neurotic defense mechanism involving avoidance of uncomfortable affect accomplished by focusing on intellectual processes.

Interpretation: a statement by the therapist that helps the patient to consciously understand the unconscious roots of a thought, feeling, or behavior. This may involve drawing a parallel between present and past experiences.

***Isolation of affect:** a neurotic defense mechanism in which an individual avoids distress by disregarding any affect related to an idea or situation.

Mentalization: the capacity to reflect on one's own mental/emotional experience and to conceptualize the different experience of another.

Negative countertransference: a therapy-contaminating emotional reaction (in the therapist) to the patient that occurs as a result of the therapist's personal issues or needs.

Neurotic personality organization: pertains to individuals who tend to view self and others as having a blend of good and bad qualities, have stable identity, possess good impulse control, have intact and stable reality testing, have a capacity for mentalization, and tend to use defenses such as repression, intellectualization, undoing, reaction formation, rationalization, displacement, and isolation of affect (Gabbard, 2004, p. 31). Despite their capacity for whole object relations, individuals with neurotic personality organization tend to be self-critical and may experience significant intrapsychic conflict and anxiety.

Object: a mental representation of oneself or another that is invested with emotional energy.

Object constancy: the capacity to maintain a stable, balanced, and accurate mental image of another.

Object relations: one of the four main theoretical frameworks of psychodynamic psychotherapy. Focuses on inaccuracies in the individual's mental representations (i.e., ways of perceiving and understanding) of self and others and the impact of these on the person's relationships.

Object representation: a mental image or way of viewing another that may or may not be accurate or realistic.

Observing ego: the part of the psyche that has the capacity to observe one's thoughts, feelings, and behavior.

Paranoid-schizoid position: an infantile state of panic driven by the fear of annihilation by a malevolent external source.

Partial object relations: the tendency to maintain unintegrated "all-good" or "all-bad" mental representations of self and others.

*Projection: an immature defense mechanism in which an individual attributes unacceptable internal thoughts or feelings to an external source.

Projective identification: an immature defense mechanism involving two steps. In the first step, one person behaves in such a way as to project an intolerable thought or feeling onto the second person. This occurs via interpersonal pressure designed to induce the second person to take on the thought or feeling. In the second step, the second person thinks, feels, and behaves as if characterized by the projected thought or feeling.

Psychic determinism: a fundamental psychodynamic concept that views every person's behavior and intrapsychic processes as inextricably linked to unconscious forces that exist as a result of past experiences.

Psychodynamic psychotherapy: encompasses therapeutic approaches that focus on conscious and unconscious forces that determine behavior, attitudes, ego function, self-concept and cohesiveness, and the quality of one's relationships. Treatment generally focuses on the exploration and analysis of defense mechanisms, transference, and resistance.

* **Rationalization:** a neurotic defense mechanism in which an individual uses rational explanation to avoid distress and justify unacceptable thoughts, feelings, or behaviors.

* **Reaction formation:** a neurotic defense mechanism in which an individual transforms an unacceptable wish into its opposite in order to avoid distress.

* **Regression:** an immature defense mechanism in which an individual returns to an earlier developmental level of functioning in order to avoid discomfort or distress at the current level.

* **Repression:** a neurotic defense mechanism in which an unacceptable thought, feeling, or wish is kept outside of conscious awareness.

Resistance: the patient's conscious and/or unconscious opposition to the treatment.

Self psychology: one of the four main theoretical frameworks of psychodynamic psychotherapy. Focuses on the importance of developing and maintaining a cohesive sense of self. Posits that individuals will seek out relationships with people who reinforce a positive and cohesive view of the self.

Self representation: a mental image or way of viewing oneself that may or may not be accurate or realistic.

* **Somatization:** an immature defense mechanism in which uncomfortable thoughts or feelings are transformed into physical symptoms.

* **Splitting:** an immature defense mechanism that reduces anxiety by keeping notions of good and bad separate in the person's mind.

* **Sublimation:** a mature defense mechanism in which an unacceptable thought, feeling, or wish is redirected into a constructive, healthy outlet.

* **Suppression:** a mature defense mechanism in which an individual makes the conscious decision to temporarily set aside an uncomfortable thought, feeling, or wish.

Glossary

Transference: the process by which a patient unconsciously and inaccurately perceives the therapist as possessing qualities that characterized important figures from her past (often a parent).

Transitional object: a blanket, toy, or other inanimate object that a child imbues with the caregiver's soothing qualities.

*****Undoing:** a neurotic defense mechanism in which an individual attempts to reverse and negate an unacceptable thought, feeling, behavior, or wish, by thinking, stating, or doing its opposite.

Whole object relations: viewing self and others in an integrated fashion in which self and others are realistically characterized by a blend of coexistent good and bad qualities.

Suggested Reading List

Bender, S., and Messner, E. (2003). *Becoming a therapist: What do I say, and why?* New York: The Guilford Press.

Cashdan, S. (1988). *Object relations therapy: Using the relationship*. New York: W. W. Norton & Company, Inc.

Ekman, P. (2003). *Emotions revealed: Recognizing faces and feelings to improve communication and emotional life*. New York: Holt Paperbacks.

Gabbard, G. O. (2004). *Long-term psychodynamic psychotherapy: A basic text*. Arlington, VA: American Psychiatric Publishing, Inc.

Gabbard, G. O. (2005). *Psychodynamic psychiatry in clinical practice*. Arlington, VA: American Psychiatric Publishing, Inc.

Hamilton, G. N. (1990). *Self and others: Object relations theory in practice*. Northvale, NJ: Jason Aronson, Inc.

McWilliams, N. (1999). *Psychoanalytic case formulation*. New York: The Guilford Press.

Pease, A., and Pease, B. (2004). *The definitive book of body language*. New York: Bantam Dell.

Shea, S. C. (1998). *Psychiatric interviewing: The art of understanding*. Philadelphia: W. B. Saunders Company.

Yalom, I. (2002). *The gift of therapy: An open letter to a new generation of therapists and their patients.* New York: HarperCollins.

Yeomans, F. E., Clarkin, J. F., and Kernberg, O. S. (2005). *A primer of transference-focused psychotherapy for the borderline patient.* Lanham, MD: Rowman & Littlefield Publishers, Inc.

Index